before the last date shown be

B

AAS
Agents and Actions Supplements
Vol. 29

Series Editor
K. Brune, Erlangen

Birkhäuser Verlag
Basel · Boston · Berlin

Risk Factors for Adverse Drug Reactions – Epidemiological Approaches

Edited by

E. Weber
D. H. Lawson
R. Hoigné

1990

Birkhäuser Verlag
Basel · Boston · Berlin

Volume Editor's Adress

Prof. E. Weber
Abt. Klinische Pharmakologie
Medizinische Universitätsklinik
Bergheimer Strasse 58
D–6900 Heidelberg 1, Fed. Rep. of Germany

This symposium was sponsored by:
Abbott, Asta Pharma, Behringwerke, Beiersdorf, Boehringer Ingelheim Fonds, Boehringer Mannheim, Byk Gulden Lomberg, Ciba-Geigy (Basel), Ciba-Geigy (Wehr), Deutsche Wellcome, Farmitalia Carlo Erba, Grünenthal, Hoechst, Hoechst UK, Henning Berlin, Hoffmann La Roche (Basel), ICI-Pharma, Kanoldt Arzneimittel, Knoll, E. Merck, Merz, Minden Pharma, Paul-Martini-Stiftung, Röhm Pharma, Sandoz (Basel), Schering, Stada Arzneimittel, The Wellcome Foundation, Dr. Willmar Schwabe

CIP-Titelaufnahme der Deutschen Bibliothek

Risk factors for adverse drug reactions – epidemiological approaches / [this symposium was sponsored by: Abbott ...].
Ed. by E. Weber ... – Basel ; Boston ; Berlin : Birkhäuser,
1990
  (Agents and actions : Supplements ; Vol. 29)
  ISBN 3-7643-2372-8 (Basel ...)
  ISBN 0-8176-2372-8 (Boston)
NE: Weber, Ellen [Hrsg.]; Agents and actions / Supplements

Product Liability: The publisher cannot assume any legal responsibility for given data, especially as far as directions for the use and the handling of drugs and chemicals are concerned. This information can be obtained from the manufacturers of drugs, chemicals and laboratory equipment.

© 1990 Birkhäuser Verlag
  P.O. Box 133
  4010 Basel
  Switzerland

Copy-Editing and layout by: Dr. J. C. F. Habicht, D–6915 Dossenheim/Heidelberg, F.R.G.

Printed in Germany on acid-free paper
ISBN 3-7643-2372-8
ISBN 0-8176-2372-8

TABLE OF CONTENTS

List of Speakers 7

Introductory remarks

E. WEBER 9

Full-length papers

Old age - is it a risk factor for
adverse drug reactions?

J. H. GURWITZ and J. AVORN 13

Gastrointestinal bleeding from the
nonsteroidal anti-inflammatory drugs

B. L. STROM, M. I. TARAGIN and J. L. CARSON 27

Time pattern of allergic reactions to drugs

R. HOIGNE, M. D'ANDREA JAEGER, R. WYMANN,
A. EGLI, U. MÜLLER, T. HESS, R. GALEAZZI,
R. MAIBACH and U. P. KÜNZI 39

Drug development optimization - benzodiazepines

M. H. LADER 59

Extrapyramidal symptoms in neuroleptic recipients

R. GROHMANN, R. KOCH and L. G. SCHMIDT 71

Epidemiological screening for potentially
carcinogenic drugs

G. D. FRIEDMAN and J. V. SELBY 83

Table of contents (continued)

Short communications

Monitoring for adverse pregnancy outcomes
related to drug exposure during pregnancy

E. ANDREWS and P. TENNIS 99

A twenty-year follow-up study on phenacetin abuse

U. C. DUBACH 101

Physician's compliance

U. C. DUBACH 103

Compliance with short-term high-dose ethinyl oestradiol in young patients with primary infertility:
new insights from the use of electronic devices

W. KRUSE, W. EGGERT-KRUSE, J. RAMPMAIER,
B. RUNNEBAUM and E. WEBER 105

Risk factors as reflected by an intensive
drug monitoring system

T. JACUBEIT, D. DRISCH and E. WEBER 117

Panel discussion

D. H. LAWSON (moderator), R. BRUPPACHER,
M. N. G. DUKES and G. R. VENNING 129

LIST OF SPEAKERS

Professor Dr. med. R. Bruppacher

Ciba-Geigy AG, P.O. Box, CH-4002 Basel, Switzerland

Professor Dr. med. U. C. Dubach

Kantonsspital Basel, Medizinische Universitäts-Polyklinik,
Petersgraben 4, CH-4031 Basel, Switzerland

Professor M. N. G. Dukes, M.D., M.A., LL.M.

World Health Organization, 8 Scherfigsvej,
DK-2100 Copenhagen, Denmark

G. D. Friedman, M.D.

The Permanente Medical Group, Inc., Division of Research,
3451 Piedmont Avenue, Oakland, CA 94611-5463, United States of America

Dr. med. R. Grohmann

Psychiatrische Klinik und Poliklinik der Universität,
Nußbaumstraße 7, D-8000 Munich, Federal Republic of Germany

J. H. Gurwitz, M.D.

Program for the Analysis of Clinical Strategies,
Harvard Medical School, Beth Israel Hospital, 333 Longwood Avenue,
Boston, MA 02115, United States of America

Professor Dr. med. R. Hoigné

Zieglerspital, Morillonstrasse, 75-91, CH-3001 Berne, Switzerland

T. Jacubeit, Assistenzärztin

Abteilung Klinische Pharmakologie, Medizinische Universitätsklinik,
Bergheimer Straße 58, D-6900 Heidelberg 1, Federal Republic of Germany

Dr. med. W. Kruse

Krankenhaus Bethanien, Rohrbacher Straße 149, D-6900 Heidelberg 1,
Federal Republic of Germany

List of speakers (continued)

Professor M. H. Lader, D.Sc., Ph.D., M.D., F.R.C. Psych.

Institute of Psychiatry, The Bethlehem Hospital and
The Maudsley Hospital, De Crespigny Park, Denmark Hill, London SE5 8AF,
United Kingdom

Professor D. H. Lawson, M.D., F.R.C.P.

Royal Infirmary, Clinical Pharmacology, Glasgow G4 OS4, United Kingdom

Professor B. L. Strom, M.D., M.P.H.

Clinical Epidemiology Unit, Section of General Internal Medicine,
University of Pennsylvania, 225L Nursing Education Building,
Philadelphia, PA 19104-6095, United States of America

P. Tennis, M.D.

Burroughs Wellcome Co., Epidemiolgy, Information & Surveillance
Division, 3030 Cornwallis Road, Research Triangle Park, NC 227709,
United States of America

Dr. G. R. Venning, M.A., B.M., F.R.C.P.

Pharmaceutical Research Services Ltd., 14 Lucas Road, High Wycombe,
Bucks HP13 6QG, United Kingdom

Priv. Doz. Dr. med. I. Walter-Sack

Abteilung Klinische Pharmakologie, Medizinische Universitätsklinik,
Bergheimer Straße 58, D-6900 Heidelberg 1, Federal Republic of Germany

Professor Dr. med. E. Weber

Abteilung Klinische Pharmakologie, Medizinische Universitätsklinik,
Bergheimer Straße 58, D-6900 Heidelberg 1, Federal Republic of Germany

INTRODUCTORY REMARKS

E. Weber

Dear colleagues,

On behalf of my fellow organizers, Professor Lawson and Professor Hoigné, and Doctor Walter-Sack, I have the great honour and pleasure of welcoming you to this satellite symposium of the Fourth World Conference on Clinical Pharmacology and Therapeutics, the CPT 89 (Mannheim/Heidelberg, 23-28 July 1989).

Seeing that the main part of the meeting ended just yesterday, we will presumably be considered to be not only workoholics but "congressoholics", as well. But then, we wanted to make sure that you would be spending at least one day in Heidelberg, and it will be our great pleasure to show you the splendours of the city on a boat tour on the Neckar this evening.

The motive for organizing this symposium was that we wanted to seize the opportunity of bringing together all fellow researchers who convened for the CPT 89 and were interested in discussing the topic. Thank you very much for being here today and for showing interest in a field where, we believe, not enough research work is being done.

The various aspects of today's subject-matter markedly reflect the multiplicity of relevant factors. Or course, we do not claim - not least for lack of time - to have covered all factors at length.

It is our aim to focus on at least some of the factors which possibly constitute important risks for adverse drugs reactions, for instance the early and late stages of life - infancy and old age; the factor of time, which so far has received too little attention; the risks connected with frequently prescribed drugs, such as the non-steroidal anti-inflammatory drugs, benzodiazepines and neuroleptics. Other risk factors, however, which are iatrogenic or due to patients' noncompliance, are also to be addressed. Finally, there will be a panel discussion on the critical subject of how the various parties involved, i.e. industry, academia and the regulatory authorities, can and do react to alleged risks.

My fellow organizers and I sincerely hope you will enjoy this symposium and that we will have met your expectations in full.

Heidelberg, 29 July, 1989

FULL-LENGTH   PAPERS

AAS 29:
Risk Factors for
Adverse Drug Reactions

OLD AGE - IS IT
A RISK FOR ADVERSE DRUG REACTIONS?

J. H. Gurwitz and J. Avorn

Abstract

Pharmacotherapy is often the single most important medical intervention in the care of the elderly. However, there are obvious concerns about the vulnerability of this group to adverse drug reactions (ADRs). A rapidly accumulating literature regarding changes in pharmacokinetics and pharmacodynamics with advancing age suggests a strong pharmacologic basis for such concerns. Yet, the results of epidemiologic studies exploring the relationship between age and ADRs are ambiguous.

Interpretation of the results of these studies is limited by inconsistent definitions of outcomes of interest and failure to control for important age-related covariates including the clinical status of the patient and the number of medications that a patient is receiving. Some recent studies have investigated age-related aspects of specific adverse consequences of drug therapy. For example, age, in and of itself, does not appear to be a risk factor for bleeding complications of warfarin therapy. Older patients may actually be at less risk than younger patients to experience depression associated with beta-blocker therapy.

Although examination of data from premarketing studies might be considered a promising strategy to explore the relationship between age and ADR risk, the small number of truly elderly subjects included in these studies greatly limits their usefulness. Postmarketing studies utilizing databases containing clinical data for large numbers of older patients may provide the optimal approach for investigating whether old age is an independent risk factor for ADRs.

Introduction

One of the main intellectual agendas for geriatrics and gerontology has been the separation of changes seen with old age, those caused by the aging process itself, and events spuriously linked to aging which, when properly studied prove to be independent of it altogether. While chronologic age often has been considered a risk factor for the occurrence of adverse drug reactions (ADRs), the relative importance of age as a valid predictor continues to be debated. Such controversy is similar to the confusion surrounding the relationship between patient age and medication compliance. While a variety of factors have been suggested as predisposing the elderly to noncompliance, the literature does not support a strong association between patient age and compliance (Darnell et al., 1986; Spagnoli et al., 1989). The present review will examine the relationship between patient age and risk of ADRs across a wide range of perspectives from the pharmacology and physiology of aging to selected epidemiologic studies which have addressed this question.

Physiology and pharmacology of aging

Cross-sectional and longitudinal studies involving community-dwelling populations indicate that increasing age is often (but not invariably) accompanied by reductions in the physiologic reserve of many organ systems, reductions that are separate from the effects of disease. Although these changes are characterized by substantial variability from individual to individual, they place many elderly individuals at special risk for morbidity from coincident insults such as infection or injury. It follows that these decrements might translate into an increased risk of ADRs in elderly patients.

Changes in pharmacokinetics and pharmacodynamics that occur with advancing age provide an additional theoretical basis for concern about ADRs in the old. Of the four traditional components of pharmacokinetics - absorption, distribution, metabolism, and excretion - only absorption appears to be substantially independent of age (Johnson et al., 1985). For certain medications, drug distribution can vary importantly in the elderly. An age-related increase in body fat at the expense of muscle leads to a greater volume of distribution and drug half-life for highly lipid-soluble medications such as the long-acting benzodiazepine hypnotics. Important pathways of drug metabolism in the liver may be impaired in advanced age (Greenblatt et al., 1982). Drug excretion by the kidney may be considerably prolonged in elderly patients due to age-related declines in renal function, although the variability of deterioration is large between individuals (Rowe et al., 1976).

For reasons that are not completely understood, the aging process appears to be associated with an increase in the sensitivity of receptors for many medications commonly prescribed to the elderly. One of the first studies describing such changes involved a sample of patients between the ages of 30 and 90 years undergoing elective cardioversion, who were medicated with diazepam (Reidenberg et al., 1976). The clinical end-point used was the patient's inability to respond to vocal stimuli, with preservation of response to a painful stimulus. The serum level of diazepam at which this effect occurred was significantly lower in elderly patients. Similar findings have emerged from studies involving other benzodiazepines and the opiates (Greenblatt et al., 1977; Bellville et al., 1971; Kaiko, 1980; Scott & Stanski, 1987). Such changes in pharmacodynamics, together with age-related changes in drug disposition, could well be expected to place the elderly patient at some increased risk for ADRs. However, this issue is not as straightforward as it would seem.

Definition of an ADR

The evaluation of the literature regarding ADRs is difficult for a number of reasons. Foremost among them is a lack of consistency in the definition employed for the outcome of interest. As pointed out by

J. H. Gurwitz and J. Avorn

Karch and Lasagna (1975), in the broadest sense, an ADR is any undesirable effect produced by a drug. Most of the studies included in the
present review have utilized this definition as it stands or with slight
modifications. Yet how this very general definition is operationalized
has important implications for the results of any study. For example,
such a definition might include the effects of intentional overdose and
drug abuse, which are not relevant to an analysis of risks associated
with the therapeutic use of medications.

General ADR studies

Over the past twenty-five years, numerous studies have explored the relationship between patient age and ADR risk (Nolan &
O'Malley, 1988). Most of these investigations involve hospital inpatient
populations. Unfortunately, the age-related analyses for many of these
studies involve crude stratifications by simple and probably inappropriate "young" versus "old" categories (e.g., patient age <65 versus ≥
65). Alternatively, the average age of patients experiencing ADRs is
compared with the average age of patients not experiencing ADRs. This
approach is likely to miss effects of aging which occur only in the very
old (i.e., over age 85). A few studies do provide adequate data to
examine age trends in the risk of ADRs (Seidl et al., 1966; Olgilvie &
Ruedy, 1967; Hurwitz, 1969; Bergman & Leaverton, 1971; Smidt & McQueen,
1972; Klein et al. 1976; Levy et al., 1977). Although the results of
these studies suggest a trend toward increasing risk with advancing age,
this conclusion is open to question because none of the reviewed investigations controlled for potentially important covariates including
clinical status, length of hospitalization, and number of medications
taken concurrently.

The unquestionable importance of controlling for relevant
covariates was confirmed by Hutchinson et al. (1986) in a study focusing upon ambulatory patients. The investigators studied 1,026 patients
seen in an internal medicine practice over a one-year period. ADRs were
detected through intensive telephone surveillance. Although the patient-
based analysis suggested a positive correlation between patient age and
the development of ADRs, when the analysis was performed examining fre-

quency of ADRs controlling for numbers of courses of drug therapy, there was no age effect.

These findings do support the obvious association between the number of drugs taken concurrently and the risk of ADRs (Williamson & Chopin, 1980; Kellaway & McGrae, 1973; Smith et al. 1966). More importantly, the number of drugs that a patient is receiving is directly related to the number of coexisting diseases (Grymonpre et al., 1988). The clinical status of a patient is one of the most important predictors of ADR risk, and the number of drugs taken concurrently is a much better proxy for the clinical status of the patient than chronologic age.

Studies of specific medications

Although many studies utilize a very general definition to describe ADRs and often combine all ADRs from all medications into a single outcome category in the analysis of predisposing factors, this should not imply that the factors leading to the occurrence of an ADR are the same in each individual patient or for each individual drug (Hurwitz, 1969). More useful information concerning the relationship between patient age and ADR risk may be derived from investigations of specific medication categories, especially when the outcome of interest is a specific type of ADR. Such studies present their own special problems in interpretation involving issues of sample size (type II error) and selection bias. However, the results of these studies provide an indication of the complexity and uncertainty surrounding the age/ADR question.

Benzodiazepine hypnotics - flurazepam

In 1987, flurazepam was the second most commonly prescribed benzodiazepine hypnotic among hospitalized patients in the U.S. (Tomita et al, 1988). The major metabolite of flurazepam, N-desalkylflurazepam, is active and has an exceedingly long half-life: 74 hours in young males and 160 hours in elderly males (Greenblatt et al., 1981).

In a landmark paper, Greenblatt et al. (1977) assessed the hazards of flurazepam in hospitalized medical patients. This report was

based upon data accumulated by the Boston Collaborative Drug Surveillance Program between 1970 and 1975 on 2,542 patients who received
flurazepam during a hospitalization. Nearly all ADRs to flurazepam were
found to involve excess central nervous system effects (excessive
drowsiness, confusion, ataxia). The authors reported that the frequency
of flurazepam ADRs increased significantly with patient age and average
daily dose. When stratifications were performed simultaneously according
to patient age and daily dose, the effect of age was noted to be striking at higher daily doses (≥ 30 mg per day), but at average daily doses
under 15 mg per day there was only a slight increase in toxicity with
advancing age (Figure 1).

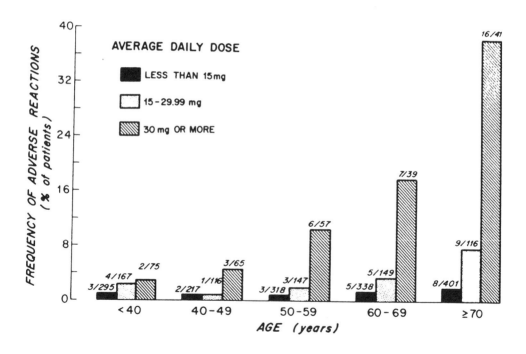

Figure 1: Frequency of adverse reactions to the benzodiazepine, flurazepam, in relation to age and drug dosage (Greenblatt et al., 1977).

Oral anticoagulant therapy

Anticoagulant therapy with warfarin sodium is critical to the optimal management of various thromboembolic and vascular disorders, which are of increasing prevalence in the elderly. In a retrospective follow-up study of 321 patients followed in an outpatient anticoagulation clinic, Gurwitz et al. (1988) evaluated the relationship between patient age and the risk of bleeding complications associated with long-term oral anticoagulant therapy. Utilizing a life-table approach to control for varying lengths of patient follow-up, no significant differences in the risk of initial minor or major bleeding complications were detected between the various age groups examined (<50, 50-59, 60-69, and $\geq$70 years) (Figures 2 and 3). Controlling for several potentially confounding factors including total number of medical problems, total number of medications, and prior warfarin exposure did not alter the results. There are important limitations to this study in terms of sample size as well as the potential for selection bias; however, its findings are in agreement with the results of an earlier investigation which utilized a similar analytic approach in a different clinical setting (Petitti et al., 1986).

Beta-blocker therapy and depression

In a population-based study less open to criticism concerning selection bias, Avorn et al. (1986) examined the association between beta-blocker therapy and depression. This investigation made use of Medicaid prescribing records to study the association of depression with the use of beta-blockers. The occurrence of depression was estimated by measuring use of tricyclic antidepressants. Among a large study sample (N=143,253), 23% of patients using beta-blockers were prescribed a tricyclic antidepressant as compared with 10% of patients taking methyldopa or reserpine, 15% taking hydralazine, and 17% taking hydrochlorothiazide. Of particular relevance to the present review, the magnitude of the association between beta-blocker and tricyclic antidepressant use was found to decline with advancing age (Figure 4). This observation probably did not result from physician reluctance to prescribe tricyclic antidepressants to older patients, since baseline use of tricyclic anti-

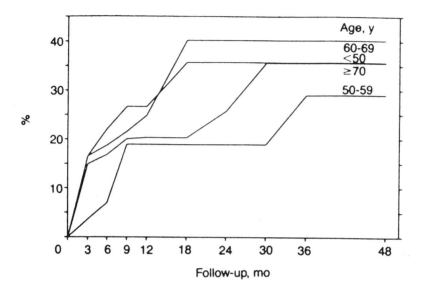

Figure 2: Risk of minor complications according to duration of long-term anticoagulant therapy and age (Gurwitz et al., 1988).

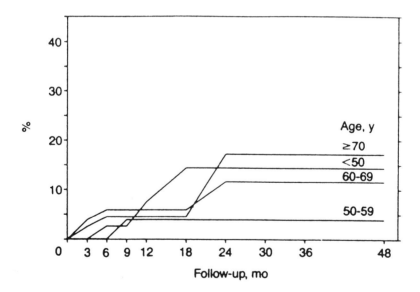

Figure 3: Risk of major bleeding complications according to duration of long-term oral anticoagulant therapy (Gurwitz et al., 1988).

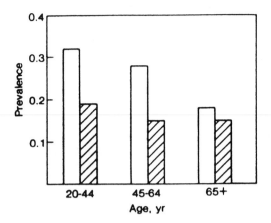

Figure 4: Antidepressant use among patients receiving beta-blockers. 2-year prevalence by age. White bars indicate women; shlashed bars, men.

depressants among older patients was controlled for relative to younger patients. Among the possible explanations for these findings, the authors speculated that central nervous system side effects of beta-blockers might be milder in older patients as compared to younger ones, consistent with pharmacodynamic studies documenting diminished sensitivity of beta-adrenergic receptor sites in old versus young subjects (Vestal et al., 1979).

Directions for future research

Premarketing studies

The analysis of data collected in premarketing drug studies would seem to be an attractive approach to elucidating the effect of age on the occurrence of ADRs. Unfortunately, there are multiple problems associated with this approach. Premarketing clinical trials often include only a modest number of elderly subjects relative to the patient population likely to be exposed to a drug once it is in widespread use.

The oldest old are generally excluded from participation in trials of investigational drugs, and elderly subjects who do participate in such trials tend to be especially healthy "young-old". These subjects may have limited generalizability to the multiply impaired older patient taking multiple medications.

The nonsteroidal anti-inflammatory drugs (NSAIDs) provide a good example of the limits of premarketing data for exploring age-related questions. For example, only 3.1 percent of over 2,000 subjects in the new drug application for the NSAID, sulindac, were over age 70 (Jaffe, 1987).

Postmarketing surveillance studies

One promising approach to the study of ADRs in the elderly involves the use of large clinical databases which incorporate patient-specific information regarding medication use linked to diagnostic information and data concerning hospitalizations and physician encounters. For example, in the U.S., over 20 million people are covered by various state Medicaid programs and most states maintain detailed computerized records of all reimbursed health care encounters on a recipient-specific basis. Such claims databases are a source of information regarding large numbers of elderly patients. These patients are likely to be more representative of the older population seen in the community than elderly subjects presently included in premarketing studies.

Several research groups have begun to report descriptive and analytic epidemiologic studies of adverse effects of medication use utilizing computerized databases. These include a description of concurrent use of multiple anticholinergic drugs in nursing home patients (Blazer et al., 1983), a cross-sectional investigation suggesting increased use of antidepressants among patients taking beta-blockers (Avorn et al., 1986) a case-control study of the role psychotropic drugs play in the risk of hip fracture (Ray et al., 1987), and a number of analyses examining the relationship between NSAID exposure and upper gastrointestinal hemorrhage (Carson et al., 1987; Carson et al., 1987a). These initial efforts serve to encourage future research endeavors which employ health care claims databases in the investigation of potential risk factors for the occurrence of ADRs.

Conclusions

This review has summarized a modest, but growing literature regarding the relationship of advanced age to the occurrence of ADRs. These investigations reflect an increasing appreciation of the importance of this issue to the optimal care of older patients. While the data presented often seem contradictory, this observation most likely reflects an emerging principle of geriatric pharmacology: individual physiologic parameters are far more important than any chronologic measure in determining whether an individual patient will tolerate a prescribed medication. Chronologic age serves as a useful predictor only so far as it reflects the physiologic status of the population one is studying. While the information and experience gained from these studies can help guide pharmacotherapeutic decision-making in the older patient, the limits of our research efforts to date must be recognized.

Acknowledgments

This work was supported in part by a grant from the John A. Hartford Foundation. Dr. Gurwitz is a Merck Fellow in Geriatric Clinical Pharmacology. The authors are grateful to Jason Bromberg and Barbara Arsenault for assistance with the preparation of the manuscript.

J. H. Gurwitz and J. Avorn

References

1. Avorn, J., Everitt, D.E., and Weiss, S. (1986) J. Am. Med. Assoc. 255, 357-360.

2. Bellville, J.W., Forrest, W.H., Miller, E., et al. (1971) J. Am. Med. Assoc. 217, 1835-1841.

3. Bergman, H.D., Leaverton, P.E. (1971) Am. J. Hosp. Pharm. 28, 343-350.

4. Blazer, D.G., Federspiel, C.F., Ray, W.A., et al. (1983) J. Gerontol. 38, 31-35.

5. Carson, J.L., Strom, B.L., Morse, M.L., et al. (1987) Arch. Intern. Med. 147, 1054-1059.

6. Carson, J.L., Strom, B.L., Soper, K.A., et al. (1987a) Arch. Intern. Med. 147, 85-88.

7. Darnell, J.C., Murray, M.D., Martz, B.L., et al. (1986) J. Am. Geriatr. Soc. 34, 1-4.

8. Greenblatt, D.J., Allen, M.D., and Shader, R.I. (1977) Clin. Pharmacol. Ther. 21, 355-361.

9. Greenblatt, D.J., Divoll, M., Harmatz, J.S., et al. (1981) Clin. Pharmacol. Ther. 30, 475-486.

10. Greenblatt, D.J., Sellers, E.M., and Shader, R.I. (1982) New Engl. J. Med. 306, 1081-88.

11. Grymonpre, R.E., Mitenko, P.A., Sitar, D.S., et al. (1988) J. Am. Geriatric Soc. 36, 1092-1098.

12. Gurwitz, J.H., Goldberg, R.J., Holden, A., et al. (1988) Arch. Intern. Med. 148, 1733-1736.

13. Hurwitz, N. (1969) Brit. Med. J. 1, 536-539.

14. Hutchinson, T.A., Flegel, K.M., Kramer, M.S., et al. (1986) J. Chron. Dis. 39, 533-42.

15. Jaffe, M.E. (1987) Clin. Pharmacol. Ther. 42, 686-92.

16. Johnson, S.L., Mayersohn, M., and Conrad, K.A. (1985) Clin. Pharmacol. Ther. 38, 331-335.

17. Kaiko, R.F. (1980) Clin. Pharmacol. Ther. 28, 823-826.

18. Karch, F.E., and Lasagna, L. (1975) J. Am. Med. Assoc. 234, 1236-1241.

19. Kellaway, G.S.M., and McCrae, E. (1973) NZ Med. J. 78, 525-528.

20. Klein, U., Klein, M., Rothenbuhler, M., et al. (1976) Int. J. Clin. Pharmacol. 13, 187-195.

21. Levy, M., Kletter-Hemo, D., Nir, I., et al. (1977) Israel J. Med. Sci. 13, 1065-1071.

22. Nolan, L., and O'Malley, K (1988) J. Am. Geriatr. Soc. 36, 142-149.

23. Olgilvie, R.I., and Ruedy, J. (1967) Canad. Med. Ass. J. 97, 1450-1457.

24. Petitti, D.B., Strom, B.L., and Melmon, K.L. (1986) Amer. J. Med. 81, 255-259.

25. Ray, W.A., Griffin, M.R., Schaffner, W., et al. (1987) N. Engl. J. Med. 316, 363-369.

26. Reidenberg, M.M., Levy, M., Warner, H., et al. (1978) Clin. Pharmacol. Ther. 23, 371-4.

27. Rowe, J.W., Andres, R., Tobin, J.D., et al. (1976) J. Gerontol. 31, 155-163.

28. Scott, J.C., and Stanski, D.R. (1987) J. Pharmacol. Exp. Ther. 240, 159-166.

29. Seidl, L.G., Thornton, G.F., Smith, J.W., et al. (1966) J. Amer. Geriatric Soc. 119, 299-315.

30. Smidt, N.A., and McQueen, E.G. (1972) NZ Med. J. 76, 397-401.

31. Smith, J.W., Seidl, L.G., and Cluff, L.E. (1966) Ann. Int. Med. 65, 629-640.

32. Spagnoli, A., Ostino, G., Borga, A.D., et al. (1989) J. Am. Geriatr. Soc. 37, 619-624.

33. Tomita, D.K., Baum, C., Kennedy, D.L., et al. (1988) Drug utilization in the United States: 1987. Ninth Annual Review. Department of Health and Human Services, Public Health Service, Food and Drug Administration, Center for Drug Evaluation and Research, Office of Epidemiology and Biostatistics.

34. Vestal, R.E., Wood, A.J.J., and Shand, D.G. (1979) Clin. Pharmacol. Ther. 26, 181-6.

35. Williamson, J., and Chopin, J.M. (1980) Age and Ageing 9. 73-80.

AAS 29:
Risk Factors for
Adverse Drug Reactions
© 1990 Birkhäuser Verlag Basel

GASTROINTESTINAL BLEEDING FROM THE
NONSTEROIDAL ANTI-INFLAMMATORY DRUGS

B.L. Strom, M.I. Taragin and J.L. Carson

Abstract

Nonsteroidal anti-inflammatory drugs (NSAIDs) represent a remarkably frequently used class of drugs. The major motivation for the use of these drugs is the known gastrointestinal (GI) toxicity of aspirin. From premarketing studies it was known that NSAIDs could cause subclinical GI bleeding, but there were no controlled studies of the association between NSAID use and clinically apparent upper GI bleeding. In part because of the frequent use of these drugs and in part because of the potential seriousness of this adverse reaction, this association has been the subject of a considerable amount of postmarketing pharmaco-epidemiology research. Despite this, many questions remain unanswered. This paper reviews the existing data on GI bleeding from NSAIDs and provides suggestions for future studies which could address some of the deficiencies in the data.

Introduction

Nonsteroidal anti-inflammatory drugs (NSAIDs) are very commonly used. The major motivation for the use of these drugs is the known gastrointestinal (GI) toxicity of aspirin. From premarketing studies, it was known that NSAIDs could cause subclinical GI bleeding, but there were no controlled studies of the association between NSAID use and clinically apparent upper gastrointestinal bleeding. In part because of the frequent use of these drugs and in part because of the potential seriousness of this adverse reaction, this association has recently been the subject of a considerable amount of postmarketing pharmacoepidemiology research. Despite this, many questions remain unanswered. This paper will review the existing data on GI bleeding and peptic ulcer from NSAIDs, along with its deficiencies, and provide suggestions for future studies which could address some of these problems.

Even with an outcome as explicit as GI bleeding, different studies can use different measures of the same outcome. In particular, GI bleeding could be assessed by the use of endoscopic abnormalities, chromium-labelled red blood cells, stool testing for occult blood, the presence or absence of visible blood, hospitalization for GI bleeding, the need for a blood transfusion, etc. We will restrict the discussion in this paper to clinically apparent GI bleeding and peptic ulcer disease, as it is unclear whether studies using the more sensitive measures of subclinical bleeding, e.g., chromium-labelled red blood cells and endoscopy, provide information useful for making conclusions about clinically meaningful disease.

Risk of UGI bleeding from NSAIDs in general

Case-control studies

There have been two case-control studies published examining the risk of GI bleeding of any type from NSAIDs in general (Table 1). The first was published by Bartle et al. (1986) and compared 57 cases of GI bleeding to 123 age- and sex-matched controls. Half of the controls were hospitalized medical patients and the other half were hospital visitors. Exposure to an NSAID was associated with an approximately four-fold increase in the risk of GI bleeding. The second was published by Levy et al. (1988) using a hospital-based surveillance system, and compared 57 patients with hematemesis or melena to 2,417 patients admitted to the hospital with conditions thought to be independent of antecedent analgesic use. After adjustments for age, sex, smoking, aspirin intake, alcohol use, and coffee consumption, the use of NSAIDs was associated with a nine-fold increased risk of GI bleeding.

Both of these studies obtained their drug exposure data by interview. Given the expectation that NSAIDs would be associated with UGI bleeding, this results in a potential for a considerable recall bias. In addition, Bartle did not control for a number of potentially important confounding variables, and excluded from the controls, but not

Table 1: Case-control studies: upper gastrointestinal bleeding and/or peptic ulcer associated with the use of nonsteroidal anti-inflammatory drugs.

Authors	Year	Study outcome	Odds ratio or relative risk (95% confidence interval)	
Bartle et al.	1986	UGI bleeding	4.3	(1.5-11.6)
Levy et al.	1988	UGI bleeding	9.1	(2.1-31)
Somerville et al.	1986	Bleeding peptic ulcer[1]	2.7	(1.7- 4.4)[2]
			3.8	(22 -64)[3]
Duggan et al.	1986	Peptic ulcer	5.0	(1.4-26.9)
Clinch et al.	1987	Peptic ulcer[1]	6.7	(6.7-12.8)
Griffin et al.	1988	Fatal peptic ulcer[1]	4.7	(3.1- 7.2)
Collier & Pain	1985	Peptic ulcer	2.3	(0.8- 6.0)[4]
		perforation	11.5	(5.8-21.3)[5]
Armstrong & Blower	1987	Life-threatening peptic ulcer disease	13.9	(9.9-18.9)

1 study restricted to elderly

2 hospital controls

3 community controls

4 patients >65 years old

5 all patients <75 years old with a negative past history for GI disease

the cases, patients with a past history of peptic ulcer disease or use of anticoagulants within the previous two months. Controls, but not cases, needed to have been seen by a physician within the previous two months. Levy was restricted to those who had no predisposing condition for GI bleeding. Compared with a group with a very low baseline risk of bleeding, the increased risk of bleeding induced by NSAIDs could indeed appear larger than it would be compared to a general population.

Somerville and associates (1986) published a case-control study comparing 230 patients over age 60 who had been hospitalized with a bleeding peptic ulcer to hospital controls and community controls matched for age and sex. The use of NSAIDs was associated with approximately a three-fold increase in risk. As with the Bartle study (1986), above, this study suffered from poor control of confounding and the possibility of recall bias.

Two case-control studies have been published examining the association between NSAID use and peptic ulcer disease, with or without UGI bleeding. Duggan et al. (1986) found a five-fold increase in risk. Clinch et al. (1987), found an almost seven-fold increased risk. Both of these studies also suffered from the possibility of recall bias, since the exposure data were collected retrospectively, as well as detection bias, since the presence of NSAID exposure may have led to more aggressive evaluation.

Griffin et al. (1988) published a case-control study investigating the association between NSAID use and fatal peptic ulcer in Medicaid patients over age 60. Controls were matched for age, sex, race, calendar year, and nursing home status, and the use of NSAIDs was associated with an almost five-fold increase in risk. Because the study used claims data to determine exposure status, it was not subject to recall bias or detection bias. However, it is unclear whether the investigators' adjustments for severity of illness and alcohol use was adequate. Also, it is likely that many cases were missed, since cases were identified via death certificates only. Finally, studies of fatal peptic ulcer are problematic, as most patients with peptic ulcer or GI bleeding do not die from these conditions. Thus, one cannot differentiate how much of this increased risk is due to NSAID-induced peptic ulcer disease and how much is due to confounding by the underlying condition which led to the patient dying from a disease which is not usually fatal.

Collier et al. (1985) published a case-control study comparing 269 cases with perforated peptic ulcer to an equal number of controls admitted to the hospital for other surgical emergencies, matched for age, sex, and date of admission. A two-fold increased risk, which was not statistically significant, was found for those less than age 65. In contrast, those over age 65 using NSAIDs were 11.5 times more likely to suffer a perforated peptic ulcer than younger individuals.

Finally, Armstrong and Blower (1987) published a case-control study of life threatening complications of peptic ulcer disease, defined as causing death or requiring emergency surgery. Of the 235 cases, 141 used NSAIDs, resulting in a 14-fold increased risk. Drug history was obtained from retrospective interview or general practitioner records. In addition to the possibility of recall bias, no attempt was made to exclude from the control group individuals whose disease could be related to NSAID use, nor to control for any differences in potential confounding variables, such as underlying illnesses or even age and sex.

Cohort studies

In contrast, the four available cohort studies showed a smaller increase in risk (Table 2). Carson et al. (1987a) published a retrospective cohort study of Medicaid patients and found a 50% increase in the risk of UGI bleeding in NSAID users. A linear dose-response relationship was found, as well as a quadratic duration-response relationship, with a steadily increasing risk for the first through fourth prescription followed by a steadily decreasing risk. This study was limited by its use of unvalidated diagnoses of gastrointestinal bleeding.

Beard et al. (1987) published a similar study using data from the Group Health Cooperative of Puget Sound. Their study was restricted to those over age 64. Their results were very similar although, with a smaller sample size, they did not quite reach statistical significance.

Guess et al. (1988) published a cohort study using data from the Saskatchewan Health Plan to explore the association between NSAIDs and fatal UGI bleeding or perforation. NSAID users aged less than 75 had a three-fold increased risk vs. non-users of similar age, which was not statistically significant. Those over age 75 had a statistically significant five-fold elevation of risk. As with the study by Griffin and associates (1988), however, a study of fatal UGI bleeding is inherently problematic.

Finally, Jick et al. (1987) examined the risk of peptic ulcer perforation from NSAIDs using data from Group Health Cooperative of Puget Sound. The relative risk was 1.6, but it was not statistically significant, presumably because of small sample size.

Table 2: Cohort studies: upper gastrointestinal bleeding and/or peptic ulcer associated with the use of nonsteroidal anti-inflammatory drugs.

Authors	Year	Study outcome	Odds ratio or relative risk (95% confidence interval)	
Carson et al.	1987a	UGI bleeding	1.5	(1.2- 2.0)
Beard et al.	1987	UGI bleeding[1]	1.4	(0.9- 2.1)
Guess et al.	1988	Fatal UGI bleeding or		
		perforation	3.1	(0.1-23.2)[2]
			5.3	(1.6-17.4)[3]
Jick et al.	1987	Peptic ulcer perforation	1.6	(0.7- 3.7)

1 study restricted to elderly

2 female patients <75 years old with a negative past history for GI disease

3 female patients >75 years old with a negative past history for GI disease

Relative gastrointestinal toxicity among NSAIDs

Determining the comparative gastrointestinal toxicity of the different NSAIDs represents an even more difficult problem. As one divides the cohort of NSAID-exposed patients into subsets of those exposed to each of the different NSAIDs, the available sample size is reduced dramatically. Yet, one is looking for differences which are quite likely to be smaller than those between NSAID-exposed patients vs. unexposed patients. Recall bias is much less of an issue, as it is less likely that one of the NSAIDs will be remembered differently from others. However, a selection bias remains a possibility, as physicians may tend to choose one drug over others for patients at higher risk of GI toxicity. In particular, a newer drug may be used in patients who had problems with older drugs.

Several groups have compared among the NSAIDs using data from spontaneous reporting systems. The United Kingdom's Committee on Safety of Medicines explored the serious GI adverse reactions reported to the UK's Yellow Card System among patients receiving NSAIDs (C.S.M. Update, 1986). Among those NSAIDs on the UK market as of 1986, they concluded the overall gastrointestinal safety of the drugs could not be distinguished, with the exception of low dose ibuprofen, which appeared to be the least toxic. Rossi et al. (1987) explored data from the US spontaneous reporting system similarly, in response to an unpublished analysis of the same data suggesting that piroxicam was associated with a higher risk of serious gastrointestinal toxicity than the other NSAIDs. After adjusting for multiple factors, including age, year, and time since marketing, they concluded that there is probably no important difference in the rate of reported gastrointestinal side effects among the NSAIDs. All these studies obviously suffer from the usual problems of spontaneous reporting systems, which are not very useful for comparing among different drugs.

Collier et al. (1986) compared the distribution of NSAID exposure among cases with hospitalized upper gastrointestinal adverse reactions vs. the market share of each NSAID. Their analyses suggested that piroxicam was the most toxic of the NSAIDs. In contrast, Biour et al. (1987) performed a similar analysis of patients admitted to an intensive care unit with gastrointestinal bleeding requiring at least three units of blood and endoscopy which confirmed a bleeding ulcer in two hospitals in Paris. They found intramuscular ketoprofen, piroxicam suppositories, and niflumic acid suppositories to pose the greatest risk, while piroxicam tablets, diclofenac, and ketoprofen posed the least risk.

Several studies have examined the frequency of gastrointestinal side effects using published randomized clinical trials (Pemberton &

Strand, 1979; Coles et al., 1983; Heller et al., 1985). No consistent difference among the NSAIDs was noted.

Inman (1985) studied perforated ulcer and gastrointestinal hemorrhage among 55,642 patients using benoxaprofen, fenbufen, zome-pirac, piroxicam, or indomethacin who had been investigated using the Prescription Event Monitoring system. No differences were found among the NSAIDs.

Carson et al. (1987) published a paper reporting on a retro-spective cohort study including 88,000 Medicaid patients dispensed one of seven NSAIDs. There was a highly significant difference among the rates of UGI bleeding associated with the use of the different NSAIDs. In particular, sulindac had a higher risk of UGI bleeding associated with its use than the other NSAIDs. When the analysis was restricted to hospitalizations for UGI bleeding, the risks associated with sulindac, vs. ibuprofen, increased from 1.7 to 2.7. These findings persisted in a separate re-analysis of 1982 data. Importantly, analyses of the average daily dose of drug dispensed compared to the maximum recommended daily dose suggested that sulindac was used in higher doses than the other drugs, a potential explanation for these findings.

Finally, Beard et al. (1987), using data from Group Health Cooperative, found no differences among elderly using different NSAIDs in their risk of UGI bleeding. Guess et al. (1988) found similar results regarding fatal gastrointestinal bleeding in Saskatchewan. However, both of these studies had sample sizes much too small to address this ques-tion validly.

Synthesis of available information

It is clear that users of NSAIDs have an increased risk of UGI bleeding compared to non-users. The magnitude of this increased risk is less certain. Cohort studies seem to suggest a modest increase only, while case-control studies suggest a larger increase. These differences may be due to misclassification bias in the cohort studies, which used automated data bases, and/or recall bias in the case-control studies, which gathered their exposure data retrospectively.

It appears that increasing age, male gender, use of alcohol, use of anticoagulants, and pre-existing abdominal conditions are independently associated with an increased risk of UGI bleeding. Data from the Collier (1985) case-control study on peptic ulcer perforation and the Guess (1988) cohort study on fatal UGI bleeding or perforation suggest that the risk of these outcomes, at least, from NSAIDs is greater in the elderly than in younger individuals. In contrast, Carson et al. (1987a) did not observe a statistically significant interaction between age and NSAIDs in their effects on UGI bleeding. It also appears clear that there is a dose-response relationship between the use of NSAIDs and UGI bleeding, and there is a suggestion of a possible quadratic duration-response relationship (Carson et al., 1987).

As to a comparison of the risk of UGI bleeding among the NSAIDs, the available data do not provide a consistent answer. The largest study performed to date suggested that use of sulindac might be associated with a higher risk than use of the other NSAIDs, perhaps due to the use of a higher average daily dose (Carson et al., 1987). Although this was reproduced twice within that study, it has not been confirmed in other studies. However, the other studies were much too small to detect a difference in risk among the NSAIDs. It is not clear whether the difference in results is only due to this and/or because the difference in dose observed in the first study was not present in the latter studies and/or because there was some other bias present in that first study. In addition, that first study involved the use of an automated data base and did not include validation of the outcomes with primary medical records. While this problem was partially mitigated by analyses restricted to inpatients, which showed accentuated differences, this does not address the possibility that some of the cases of "UGI" bleeding may have been lower gastrointestinal bleeding.

Thus, it is clear that many important questions about the association between NSAIDs and UGI bleeding remain to be addressed. Further studies are clearly needed. Given the major potential for important recall bias when addressing these questions using studies involving retrospectively collected exposure data, subsequent studies should probably be conducted using claims data bases. However, given the risk of a detection bias, it is important that such studies be restricted to hospitalizations for UGI bleeding only, and ideally they should stratify

B. L. Strom et al.

according to whether bleeding was sufficiently severe to require blood transfusions. Given the risk of misclassification bias inherent in the diagnosis data of automated data bases, particularly regarding the site of gastrointestinal bleeding, it is important that such studies be restricted to cases for whom medical records can be obtained and reviewed. In addition, close attention needs to be paid to the numerous variables which could confound or modify the effect of NSAIDs on UGI bleeding. Such studies need to be large enough to be certain that they can compare among the NSAIDs and have adequate power to perform the subgroup analyses necessary to address the many remaining questions. Other questions which should be addressed include dose-response relationships, duration-response relationships, the effect of age on the risk of UGI bleeding from NSAIDs, the effect of previous abdominal conditions on the effect of NSAIDs on UGI bleeding, etc.

Acknowledgment

Our work was supported in part by grant FD-U-000079 from the Food and Drug Administration.

References

1. Armstrong, C.P., and Blower, A.L. (1987) Gut 28, 527-32.

2. Bartle, W.R., Gupta, A.K., and Lazor, J. (1986) Arch. Intern. Med. 146, 2365-7.

3. Beard, K., Walker, A.M., Perera, D.R., Jick, H. (1987) Arch. Intern. Med. 147, 1621-3.

4. Biour, M., et al. (1987) Lancet 2, 340-1.

5. Carson, J.L., Strom, B.L., Morse, M.L., et al. (1987a) Arch. Intern. Med. 147, 1054-9.

6. Carson, J.L., Strom, B.L., Soper, K.A., West, S.L., and Morse, M.L. (1987) Arch. Intern. Med. 147, 85-8.

7. Clinch, D., Banerjee, A.K., Levy, D.W., Ostick, G., and Faragher, E.B. (1987) J. R. Coll. Phys. Lond. 21, 183-7.

8. Coles, L.S., Fries, J.F., Kraines, R.G., and Roth, S.H. (1983) Am. J. Med. 74, 820-8.

9. Collier, D.S.T.J., and Pain, J.A. (1985) Gut 26, 359-63.

10. Collier, D.S.T.J., and Pain, J.A. (1986) Lancet 1, 971.

11. Committee on Safety of Medicines Update (1986) Br. Med. J. 292, 1190-1.

12. Duggan, J.M., Dobson, A.J., Johnson, H., and Fahey, P. (1986) Gut 27, 929-33.

13. Griffin, M.R., Ray, W.A., and Schaffner, W. (1988) Ann. Intern. Med. 109, 359-63.

14. Guess, H.A., West, R., Strand, L.M., et al. (1988) J. Clin. Epidemiol. 41, 35-45.

15. Heller, C.A., Ingelfinger, J.A., and Goldman, P. (1985) Pharmacotherapy 5, 30-8.

16. Inman, W.H.W. (1985) In: Prescription-Event Monitoring News, No. 3, Hamble Valley Press, Southampton, pp. 3-13.

17. Jick, S.S., Walker, A.M., Perera, D.R., and Jick, H. (1987) Lancet 2, 380-2.

18. Levy, M., Miller, D.R., Kaufman, D.W., et al. (1988) Arch. Intern. Med. 148, 281-5.

19. Pemberton, R.E., and Strand, L.J. (1979) Dig. Dis. Sci. 24, 53-63.

B. L. Strom et al.

20. Rossi, A.C., Hsu, J.P., and Faich, G.A. (1987) Br. Med. J. 294, 147-50.

21. Somerville, K., Faulkner, G., and Langman, M. (1986) Lancet 1, 462-4.

AAS 29:
Risk Factors for
Adverse Drug Reactions
© 1990 Birkhäuser Verlag Basel

TIME PATTERN OF ALLERGIC REACTIONS TO DRUGS

R. Hoigné, M. D'Andrea Jaeger, R. Wymann, A. Egli, U. Müller,
T. Hess, R. Galeazzi, R. Maibach and U.P. Künzi

Abstract

Generalized, allergic reactions to drugs show time patterns different from those based on pharmacological concepts. We distinguish three types of reactions: acute reactions (reaction time (RT): 0-60 minutes), subacute reactions (RT: 1-24 hours) and reactions of the latent type (RT: 1 day to several weeks). In this study, allergic reactions in the strict sense are supplemented by reactions considered to be based on intolerance or idiosyncrasy to aspirin, pyrazolones, paracetamol, NSAIDs, quinidine, iodine-containing contrast media and some as yet not understood reactions to local anaesthetics.

Out of a total of 23,935 drug monitoring patients with 32,317 hospitalizations in the clinical divisions of internal medicine at three Swiss hospitals during the 1974-1987 period, 951 patients with 1,040 probably or definitely drug-related events of the selected type were recorded. Ultimately, 287 patients with 310 adverse drug reactions (ADRs) fulfilled our selection criteria and were classified into six groups of syndromes (Table 1). (Of the reactions described as maculopapular rash, unspecified rash and special exanthema, only the 159 reactions from the 1985-1987 period out of a total of 889 reactions of this type observed during the whole study period were included in our secondary evaluation.)

R. Hoigné et al.

The total number of 310 reactions (100%) showed the following RT distribution: 36 (11.6%) were of the acute type, 13 (4.2%) of the latent type, 12 (3.9%) could be interpreted as two distinct possible types of reaction to different drugs, and for 3 (1.0%) reactions, the type of reaction was indeterminable. The majority of reactions, 246 (79.4%), were of the subacute type starting within 24 hours of the last drug exposure.

Among the 36 reactions of the acute type, 7 events of acute severe dyspnoea were observed which seemed to be as life-threatening as anaphylactic or anphylactoid shock.

These hospital-epidemiological data are of interest for focusing basic research and developing further principles of drug safety.

Introduction

Allergic adverse drug reactions (ADRs) and others which are not strictly pharmacological often follow time patterns which are different from pharmacological reactions in the restricted sense. Moreover, apart from a few exceptions, the syndromes and symptoms caused are different. For the treating physicians, knowledge of these facts is indispensable if an immediate decision is necessary in view of an unexpected, possibly drug-related undesirable event in a patient. Many kinds of allergy tests and approaches to verifying a patient's sensitivity to various drugs have been developed. These have, however, not been as successful, except in the case of allergic contact eczema, heamolytic anaemia and allergic reactions to penicillins (Hoigné et al., 1988a). The literature on time patterns of allergic reactions, so important for prompt decisions, is still sparse.

An early study by von Pirquet and Schick (1905) on serum sickness was limited to reactions to foreign sera and proteins and investigated neither small-molecular nor other drugs, synthetic or semisynthetic. Allergic reactions to these agents have been studied mainly in the course of the last 25 years (Hoigné, 1965; Hoigné & Däppen, 1963; Hoigné et al., 1983; Hoigné et al., 1988a and 1988b; Idsøe et al., 1969; Westerman et al., 1966).

Reaction time (RT) was defined by Mayer (1933), a dermatologist, as the period between the last exposure to an allergen and the onset of the allergic reaction.

Based on the experience with newer drugs, mainly antibiotics, we distinguish three types of allergic reactions to drugs according to their RTs (Figure 1): acute reactions (reaction time (RT): 0-60 minutes); subacute reactions (RT: 1-24 hours) and reactions of the latent type (RT: 1 day to several weeks). The second term which is important in this context is "exposure time", or "exposure period". For most considerations concerning the causality assessment of allergic phenomena, however, reaction time is more reliable a parameter than is exposure time.

Methods

Selection of patients and ADRs

At the three clinical divisions of internal medicine participating in this study (Zieglerspital, Berne (1974-1987); Anna-Seiler-Haus, Inselspital, Berne (1976-1985); Medical Clinic A, Kantonsspital, St. Gallen (1987)), 23,935 patients with 32,317 hospital admissions were registered consecutively in the years from 1974 to 1987. The "drug monitoring patient" was defined as the recipient of at least one drug during hospitalization. Patients admitted to hospital for specific hyposensitization to bee or wasp venom only were not counted as drug monitoring patients.

Out of these patients, 951 had at least one ADR (total number: 1,040) of the selected type (allergy, intolerance, idiosyncrasy and anaphylactoid reactions). The drug-relatedness of the reactions in these patients was definite or probable. The reactions occurred during hospitalization and were identified from our database.

Four hundred and ninety-four ADRs of the selected type and also of unknown mechanism were evaluated in greater detail on the basis of the patients' hospital records. They included all of the six diagnostic groups (from the 1974-1987 period) listed in Table 1, with the exception of a subgroup of Group 3 containing maculopapular rash, unspecified rash and special exanthema. Out of these, only 187 observations (all from the 1985-1987 period) were selected as a representative sample. Reactions to blood transfusions (erythrocyte or other cell sediments), blood and blood volume substitutes and local skin reactions to epicutaneously applied drugs and subcutaneously injected heparin and calcium heparinate were excluded from the study from the beginning.

In all cases of ADRs studied in greater detail, not only the definite and probable cases of drug-relatedness, but the possible ones, too, were reconsidered on the basis of the patients' hospital records. "Definite", "probable" and "possible" were defined as "proven by re-exposure", "probability of drug causality greater than that of non-drug causality" and "probabilities of drug and non-drug causality approximately equal", respectively.

Table 1: Syndrome classification: the six groups of allergic reactions to drugs, with the observed number of selected ADRs in parentheses.

---

1. Anaphylactic shock (2), anaphylactoid shock (4), acute severe dyspnoea (7) and anaphylactoid reactions (2)

2. Urticaria, angioedema (49), bronchial asthma attack (11) and drug fever (36)

3. Maculopapular rash and unspecified rash (154), special exanthemas (5), conjunctivitis (1) and vascular purpura (12)

4. Serum sickness and serum sickness syndrome (4) and allergic vasculitis, including typical cases without histological examination (12)

5. Thrombocytopenia (1), agranulocytosis and neutropenia (5), and PIE syndrome (pulmonary infiltration with eosinophilia) (2)

6. Liver (3) and kidney (0) reactions

Two hundred and eighty-seven patients with 310 ADRs satisfied our selection criteria (including 159 of all 889 reactions in the sub-group of Group 3). All events were included which were considered to be probably or definitely drug-related and involved allergy, intolerance, idiosyncrasy and anaphylactoid reactions as pathomechanism.

In spite of differing opinions in the literature, all cases of exanthema in Group 3 were attributed to the allergic mechanism (Hoigné et al., 1988a), except for those observed under aspirin, pyrazolones, paracetamol or NSAIDs, which were counted as intolerance reactions.

Reaction time

Our questionnaire, in use since 1974, does not include reaction time (RT) as an indispensable item. Therefore, RTs had to be taken from the patients' hospital records. RTs of 0-60 minutes had to be clearly stated in the records for data to be accepted in this category. Such reactions were termed acute reactions. In patients undergoing continuous drug therapy, reactions described as setting in within 6-8 hours (equivalent to 3 or 4 doses of drug per 24 hours) were considered as occurring within 0-24 hours (most probably to be interpreted as between 1 and 24 hours), i.e. as reactions of the subacute type. A number of objective signs without observed symptoms might, however, have been overlooked during the first hour. This is a problem innate in most drug monitoring methods.

The reactions considered to be of the latent type set in more than one day after the last drug exposure and generally occurred after discontinuation of the drug for reasons other than ADRs (Tables 2 & 4).

If an event was attributable to at least two different drugs, given at separate times, no decision was made as to which of the two RTs was the more likely one (Table 3). Usually, the drug with the longer reaction time rather than the one with the shorter (more common) RT is likely to be the cause of the observed syndrome.

Classification and hierarchy of syndromes

-   Fever with exanthema was counted as fever.

- Urticaria was considered to be more important than angioedema, and angioedema more important than a skin rash.
- Bronchospasm was considered to be more important than angioedema. (No case of laryngeal oedema was observed.)
- Blood dyscrasias were considered to be more important than fever or skin rashes.

Pathomechanisms

- The expressions "allergic" or "nonallergic" were used for reactions resembling Type-I immune mechanisms related to a local anaesthetic.
- The expression "anaphylactoid" was used for probably nonallergic circulatory reactions (Table 6).
- Agranulocytosis or thrombocytopenia in patients under treatment with beta-lactam antibiotics were regarded as pharmacological reactions, even in the presence of exanthema (Neftel et al., 1985; Neftel and Hübscher, 1987). With cotrimoxazole, acute agranulo- cytosis, neutropenia and thrombocytopenia were defined as allergic reactions only in patients who otherwise were in good condition and nutritional state.
- All cases of exanthema in Group 3 were attributed to the allergic mechanism, except for those under treatment with aspirin, pyrazo- lones, paracetamol or NSAIDs, which were all counted as intolerance reactions (Table 6).

Results

Out of all 23,935 patients (32,317 hospital admissions), 951 developed at least one ADR (1,040 in total) involving the following mechanisms: allergy, idiosyncrasy or intolerance, and anaphylactoid reaction. Accordingly, reactions of the selected types were seen in 3.2% of all admissions. As the overall rate of ADRs was ca. 15%, one in five patients with ADRs developed at least one reaction of the selected type.

In all 15 events involving anaphylactic or anaphylactoid shock, anaphylactoid reaction or acute severe dyspnoea, the onset of the reaction was within 60 minutes of the last drug exposure (Table 2).

Table 2: Case number analysis according to syndromes and reaction times.

Syndrome (total number of cases observed)	Reaction time (RT)				
	0-60 min	1*-24 hr	1-8 d.	2 possible RTs	indeterminable
Anaphylactic shock (2)	2	0	0	0	0
Anaphylactoid shock (4)	4	0	0	0	0
Anaphylactoid reactions (2)	2	0	0	0	0
Acute severe dyspnea (7)	7	0	0	0	0
Urticaria/angioedema (49)	10 (21%)	34 (69%)	3 (6%)	2 (4%)	0
Bronchial asthma attack (11)	7 (64%)	3 (27%)	0	0	1 (9%)
Drug fever (36)	1 (2.8%)	32 (89%)	1 (2.8%)	1 (2.8%)	1 (2.8%)
Exanthemas** (159***)	2 (1%)	143 (90%)	5 (3%)	9 (6%)	0
Rhinitis (1)	1	0	0	0	0
Vascular purpura (12)	0	11 (92%)	1 (8%)	0	0
Serum sickness and Serum sickness syndrome (4)	0	3 (75%)	1 (25%)	0	0
Allergic vasculitis (12)	0	11 (92%)	1 (8%)	0	0
Thrombocytopenia (1)	0	1	0	0	0
Agranulocyt./Neutropenia (5)	0	4 (80%)	0	0	1 (20%)
PIE syndrome (2)	0	2	0	0	0
Hepatic reactions (3)	0	2 (67%)	1 (33%)	0	0
Totals (overall: 310****)	36 (12%)	246 (79%)	13 (4%)	12 (4%)	3 (1%)

* medical records indicated no ADR symptoms up to 1 hr after administration
** maculopapular and unspecified exanthema as well as special exanthemas
*** in this subgroup of Group 3, only data from 1985-1987 were evaluated
**** %'s in this line are biased, as only a subgroup of Group 3 was included

Table 3: Reactions with two possible reaction times (RTs).

Syndrome	No. of observation, sex, year of birth	Yr. of observation	Drug	RT* I	II	III
Urticaria	1. m 1926	1985	Metamizol	x		
			Spasmo-Cibalgin comp.[R]		x (8h)	
	2. f 1909	1978	Metamizol	x		
			Toquilone comp.[R]			x
	3. f 1918	1983	Heparin	x		
			Ceftriaxone, Penicillin G			x
Maculopapular and unspecified exanthemas, and special exanthemas	4. m 1911	1987	Furosemide	x		
			Augmentin[R]			x
	5. f 1916	1985	Proprandol	x		
			Amoxicillin			x
	6. f 1932	1987	Clomethiazole	x		
			Ceftriaxone			x
	7. f 1894	1986	Metamizol	x		
			Amoxicillin			x
	8. f 1904	1985	Ranitidine	x		
			Amoxicillin			x
	9. m 1926	1985	Rifampicin	x		
			Flucloxacillin			x
	10. f 1906	1985	Paracetamol, Diclofenac	x		
			Amoxicillin			x
	11. f 1937	1985	Tamoxifen	x		
			Augmentin[R]			x
	12. f 1921	1986	Furosemide	x		
			Moduretic[R]			x

* RT: I, II and III = 0-60 min, 1-24 hrs, and 1-8 days, resp. (cf. Tab. 2)

Spasmo-Cibalgin comp.[R]: Codeine phosphate + allobarbital + hexahydroadiphenine + propyphenazone

Toquilone comp.[R]: Methaqualone + diphenhydramine

Augmentin[R]: Amoxycillin + clavulanic acid

Moduretic[R]: Hydrochlorothiazide + amiloride

Table 4: Time patterns of allergic reactions to drugs: the syndromes and their relation to drug exposure.

Syndrome	Relationship between drug exposure and ADR onset			
	1st day	during drug treatment	>24 hrs after discontinuation	indeter- minable*
Anaphylactic shock (2)	2	0	0	0
Anaphylactoid shock (4)	4	0	0	0
Anaphylactoid reactions (2)	2	0	0	0
Acute severe dyspnea (7)	4 (57%)	3 (43%)	0	0
Urticaria/angioedema (49)	12 (24.5%)	31 (63.3%)	3 (6.1%)	3 (6.1%)
Bronchial asthma attack (11)	8 (73%)	3 (27%)	0	0
Drug fever (36)	9 (25%)	25 (69%)	1 (3%)	1 (3%)
Exanthemas** (159***)	5 (3%)	138 (87%)	5 (3%)	11 (7%)
Rhinitis (1)	1	0	0	0
Vascular purpura (12)	1 (8.3%)	10 (83.3%)	1 (8.3%)	0
Serum sickness and Serum sickness syndrome (4)	0	3 (75%)	1 (25%)	0
Allergic vasculitis (12)	0	11 (92%)	1 (8%)	0
Thrombocytopenia (1)	0	1	0	0
Agranulocyt./Neutropenia (5)	0	4 (80%)	0	1 (20%)
PIE syndrome (2)	0	2	0	0
Hepatic reactions (3)	0	2 (67%)	1 (33%)	0
Totals (overall: 310)	48 (15.5%)	233 (75.2%)	13 (4.2%)	16 (5.2%)

* due to exposure to more than one drug (incl. the 12 ADRs in Tab. 3)

** maculopapular and unspecified exanthema as well as special exanthemas

*** in this subgroup of Group 3, only data from the 1985-1987 period were evaluated in detail

In addition, there were another 21 reactions of the acute (or immediate) type, bringing the total number of acute reactions up to 36. Relative to the 310 events considered, this corresponds to a rate of 11.6%. The majority of the ADRs, 246 (79.4%), were of the subacute type (onset within 24 hours of the last drug exposure), and 13 (4.0%) were of the latent type (as defined in this study, i.e. onset was 1-8 days after last exposure). For twelve (3.9%) of the ADRs there were two possible interpretations, because two different drugs were involved (Table 3), and for 3 (1.0%) ADRs, no record of the reaction time was available.

The different syndromes and time patterns of manifestations and their relation to drug exposure are shown in Table 4. They are comparable with the syndromes and reaction times given in Table 2. There is a certain relationship between the four different pathomechanisms defined above and the three types of reaction time, as shown in Table 5.

Table 5: Pathomechanisms and their relation to reaction time (RT).

Reaction time (no. of reactions)	Pathomechanisms			
	Allergic	Allergic or nonallergic*	Anaphylac- toid	Intolerance
0-60 minutes (36)	13	2	6	15
1**-24 hours (246)	227	0	0	19
24 hrs to 8 days (13)	13	0	0	0
Two possible RTs (12)	11	0	0	1
Indeterminable (3)	2	1	0	0
Total number (310)	266	3	6	35

 * reaction to anaesthetics

** medical records indicated no ADR symptoms up to 1 hr after administration

Table 6: Nonallergic pathomechanisms and the drugs connected with them.

Pathomechanism	Total no. of events	Drug involved	No. of events
Allergic or nonallergic	3	Lidocaine	2
		Mepivacaine	1
Anaphylactoid reaction	6	Bilivistan[R]*	1
		Droperidol	1
		Lidocaine	1
		Quinidine	1
		Urografin[R]*	2
Intolerance	35	Aloxiprin	1
(Idiosyncracy)		Baralgin[R]**	1
		Bilivistan[R]*	3
		Diclofenac	3
		Dicobalt edetate	1
		Dimer-X[R]*	1
		Erythrosin (colorant in erythrocin preparations)	1
		Ibuprofen	1
		Konakion[R]***	1
		Lipiodol	1
		Metamizol	6
		„ + Spasmo-Cibalgin comp.[R]****	1
		Naproxen	2
		Omnipaque[R]*	1
		Paracetamol	2
		Rayvist[R]*	1
		Telebrix[R]*	5
		Urografin[R]*	2
		Urovist[R]*	1

* iodine-containing contrast medium

** metamizol + fenpiverinium bromide + pitofenone

*** phytomenadione (probably with cremophor)

**** codeine phosphate + allobarbital + hexahydroadiphenine + propyphenazone

Discussion

The present study is based on 23,935 drug monitoring patients included in the drug monitoring programme involving 32,317 admissions to state and regional hospitals in Switzerland.

For each patient, adverse events which were at least possibly due to drug exposure and followed the mechanisms of allergy, intolerance, idiosyncrasy and anaphylactoid reactions were analysed in detail, using not only our database, which has been computerized since 1974, but also each patient's hospital record.

Syndromes

Compared with early studies from the 1960s (Hoigné, 1965; Hoigné & Däppen, 1963; Idsøe et al, 1969; Westerman et al., 1966), the syndrome of acute severe dyspnoea has been added to the acute (or immediate) reactions (anaphylactic shock; anaphylactoid shock and anaphylactoid reactions) (Figure 1 and Table 1). These reactions did not

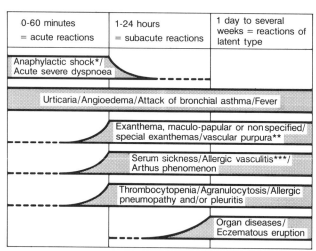

0-60 minutes = acute reactions	1-24 hours = subacute reactions	1 day to several weeks = reactions of latent type
Anaphylactic shock*/ Acute severe dyspnoea		
Urticaria/Angioedema/Attack of bronchial asthma/Fever		
	Exanthema, maculo-papular or non specified/ special exanthemas/vascular purpura**	
	Serum sickness/Allergic vasculitis***/ Arthus phenomenon	
	Thrombocytopenia/Agranulocytosis/Allergic pneumopathy and/or pleuritis	
		Organ diseases/ Eczematous eruption

* including anaphylactoid shock and anaphylactoid reactions
** without thrombocytopenia, without clinical or histological evidence of vasculitis
*** including clinically typical cases without histology

Figure 1: Reaction time and syndrome.

involve any detectable signs of bronchial obstruction; all 5 patients, with a total of 7 reactions, recovered. We do not use the term "acute respiratory distress", which was coined by Delage and Irey (1972) for a probably comparable syndrome; that term was introduced rather more in the context of traumatic shock and defined pulmonary lesions starting with oedema (Lancet Editorial, 1986).

Furthermore, in the group of patients with serum sickness and serum sickness syndrome, the diagnosis of allergic vasculitis was also accepted for typical clinical cases without performing histology. Generalized allergic vasculitis and serum sickness syndrome often appear to be two different manifestations of the same kind of disease. The term "serum sickness syndrome" was only accepted if at least three of the following symptoms, fever, arthralgia/arthritis, exanthema, leukopenia or possibly organ disease, were present at the same time (Hoigné et al., 1983).

Time patterns

Two definitions are essential for the study of drug effects and ADRs: exposure time and reaction time (Hoigné, 1965; Hoigné et al., 1983).

Exposure time has to be expressed in terms of exposure period or period of treatment and the discontinuous administration of individual doses of a drug. Generally, the manifestation of drug allergy begins only after an exposure period of at least a few days, 5-7 or more. This is the minimum time necessary for sensitization and appearance of symptoms in connection with the next dose of the drug. The first exposure in relation to a second one or a subsequent period of drug treatment is especially important in the elicitation of both anaphylactic or anaphylactoid shock (Hoigné et al., 1988b) and acute severe dyspnoea.

Single doses of drugs are mainly given in symptomatic treatment of discomfort or minor disease. With some drugs, intermittent therapy should be avoided because this may lead to an increased risk of sensitization (e.g. rifampicin/thrombocytopenia).

The rate at which exanthema occurs depends on the exposure time (Bergoend et al., 1968; Hoigné et al., 1987). In aminopenicillin-associated exanthema, the rate increases with the length of exposure, up to 12 days. In patients who have not had a skin reaction by that time, the risk per day then markedly diminishes during continued treatment (Fig. 2, Hoigné et al., 1987). This distribution pattern is not unique to the rash in patients treated with aminopenicillin preparations. Bergoend et al. (1968) reported similar findings with a long-acting sulphonamide.

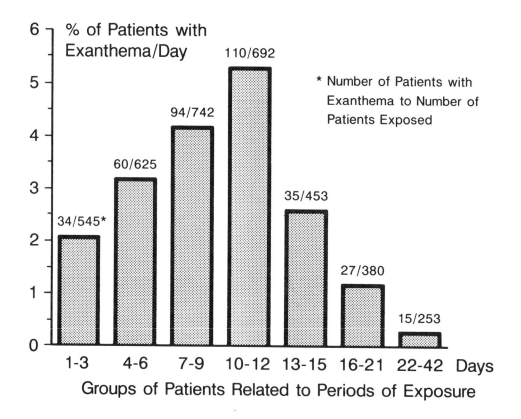

Figure 2: Relative frequency of exanthemas as a function of the periods of exposure to aminopenicillin preparations (Hoigné at al., 1987).

Reaction time, a term introduced by Mayer (1933), is the time between the last drug exposure and the appearance of the first symptoms, under the assumption of an allergic mechanism. Frequently, there is a definite relationship between the reaction time and the type of clinical syndrome. This holds true not only for reactions of the skin; as early as 1905, von Pirquet and Schick described this observation with respect to anaphylactic shock and serum sickness due to foreign sera (von Pirquet & Schick, 1905).

However, in drug allergies (involving small-molecular drugs, synthetic or semisynthetic drugs other than complete foreign antigens) much shorter reaction times are observed (Hoigné, 1965; Hoigné & Däppen, 1963; Hoigné et al., 1983, Hoigné et al., 1988a, Idsøe et al., 1969; Westerman et al., 1966).

In 1965, we proposed a new classification according to three types of reaction time: 0-60 minutes (acute reaction; some authors prefer the term "immediate reaction" (Idsøe et al., 1969; Westerman et al., 1966)), 1-24 hours (subacute reaction) and 1 day to several weeks (reaction of the latent type). This concept was advanced on the basis of 191 observations, 41 of which were made by ourselves and 150 were taken from the literature (Hoigné, 1965). Now, on the basis of our Comprehensive Hospital Drug Monitoring Program Berne/St. Gallen (CHDM), in which all patient admissions are continually registered, we have critically investigated the usefulness of this classification with respect to allergic reactions to drugs, including a number of cases of intolerance, idiosyncrasy and anaphylactoid reaction. Four hundred and ninety-four ADRs were evaluated in greater detail using the patients' hospital records (Table 1). In the case of a subgroup of skin reactions (maculo-papular rash; unspecified rash and special types of exanthema) which corresponded to the exanthema groups A and C (Hoigné et al., 1988b), only the 187 events from the 1985-1987 period out of 889 (1974-1987) were included.

With respect to the acute reactions, all instances of anaphylactic shock, anaphylactoid reactions and acute severe dyspnoea (Tables 1 and 2) followed this time pattern. Furthermore, 7 out of 10 attacks of bronchial asthma and 10 out of 49 urticarial skin reactions were also of the acute type. This finding is consistent with what one might expect for Type-I immediate allergic reactions, as defined by Coombs and Gell

R. Hoigné et al.

(1963). Out of a total of 36 reactions of the acute type, 13 were considered to be allergic, 2 were regarded as allergic or not allergic, 6 as anaphylactoid and 15 as being instances of intolerance (Table 5).

The majority of the selected reactions (246, or 79%) were of the dominant subacute type: drug fever (32), various common exanthema (143), vascular purpura (11) and allergic vasculitis (11). Urticaria was spread over all three RT categories, with 34 reactions (69.4%) belonging to the subacute type with reaction times ranging from 1-24 hours.

Latent-type reactions were observed only 13 times, or in 4% of all reactions, and included urticaria, exanthema, drug fever, vascular purpura, serum sickness (in response to horse serum), allergic vasculitis and hepatic reaction (one case). As can be seen from Table 3, 11 other reactions may have been of the latent type, but in these instances at least one additional drug had been given. Due to this fact, a second possible interpretation of these reactions arises in view of the now shorter reaction time typical of the subacute type of reaction, even though in most cases the last drug given was less known to cause the observed syndrome.

Of the 28 reactions involving vascular purpura, serum sickness or serum sickness syndrome, and allergic vasculitis, 3 (10.7%) were of the latent type. Urticaria, angioedema, vascular purpura and hepatic reaction, too, were more frequently observed in this group than were the other syndromes (Tables 2 and 4).

The total percentages given are biased due to the fact that only 159 out of 889 ADRs in the subgroup of Group 3 (Table 2) were evaluated in greater detail and included in the calculations. Assuming that all 889 ADRs have the same RT distribution as the 159 ADRs included, we can estimate the distribution for the entire 1,040 ADRs (not just for the 310). The figures then change as follows:

- acute reactions: 4.3% instead of 12%
- subacute reactions: 86.8% instead of 79%
- reactions of the latent type: 3.5% instead of 4%

Most of the concepts on which the three types of reaction time are based were confirmed by the observations presented here (Figure 1 and Table 2), with the exception of bronchial asthma attack, PIE syn-

54

drome, thrombocytopenia and agranulocytosis, which were never observed as latent type reactions in the CHDM (Table 2). Such examples are mentioned in the original literature (Hoigné, 1965), but they represent rare events.

Comparison of the three types of reaction time with the time pattern of manifestations in relation to drug exposure shows that 30 out of the 36 acute reactions started on the first day of drug administration. Probably these patients had been sensitized by previous exposure to the same drug or a chemically related one, at least in the case of anaphylactic and allergic reactions, though not necessarily in the case of anaphylactoid and intolerance reactions (comparison of Tables 2 and 4).

Furthermore, all 13 reactions of the latent type set in between 24 hours and 8 days after discontinuation of the imputed drug.

It is interesting to see that all of the 8 acute reactions with anaphylactic/anaphylactoid shock or anaphylactoid reactions (Table 2) started on the first day of drug exposure (possibly at the beginning of a new exposure period, at least as far as the allergic reactions are concerned) (Table 4).

The pathomechanisms involved were mainly chosen and assigned on the basis of modern concepts and clinical evidence, without particular investigation. It is a rather unexpected finding that out of the 36 events of the acute-reaction type only 13 satisfied the criteria of allergy, compared with 6 anaphylactoid, 15 intolerance and 2 allergic or nonallergic reactions (Tables 2 and 5).

One of the problems with these observations is the fact that syndromes and time patterns were also used to estimate the probability of drug-relatedness during primary evaluation.

In order to minimize this source of possible misinterpretation, all definite and probable ADRs, and even the possible ADRs, were reviewed in detail (secondary evaluation) using the patients' hospital records. Only "questionable" drug reactions, e.g. those not known from the literature or our own experience, were not included in our secondary evaluation. Finally, the study was restricted to reactions regarded as definitely or probably drug-related.

The drugs which were thought to play a part in nonallergic pathomechanisms of the ADRs we selected are listed in Table 6.

R. Hoigné et al.

The usefulness of the proposed classification of three clearly defined types of reaction time can be summarized from two different angles:

1. from the scientific point of view; the syndromes of a selected group of ADRs can be studied epidemiologically, irrespective of the exact pathomechanisms of the reactions. Categorization according to reaction time can serve as a further basis for more detailed and possibly bio-chemical and immunological studies on the mechanisms involved and for appropriate treatment (e.g. acute severe dyspnoea syndrome), and

2. from the clinical and the teaching point of view; the proposed clas-sification offers the possibility of a clear procedure for estimating the probability that a given event really is an ADR and, in the presence of more than one drug, it can help determine the causality of each of the drugs involved.

Acknowledgment

The CHDM Foundation is supported by the "Schweizerische Aerzteorganisation (FMH)", the "Schweizerischer Apothekerverein (SAV)" as well as Ciba-Geigy AG, Hoffmann-La Roche & Co AG and Sandoz AG, Basel, Switzerland.

References

1. Bergoend, H., Löffler, A., Amar, R., Maleville, J. (1968) Annals Derm. Syph., Paris 95, 5-6, 481-490.

2. Coombs, R.R.A., and Gell, P.G.H. (1963) The classification of allergic reactions underlying disease; In: Clinical aspects of Immunology. Chapter 13 (P.G.H. Gell and R.R.A. Coombs, Eds), Blackwell Scientific, Oxford, pp. 373-377.

3. Delage, C., Irey, N.S. (1972) J. Forens. Sci. 17, No. 4, 525-540.

4. Editorial (1986) Lancet 301-303.

5. Hoigné, R. (1965) Arzneimittelallergien. Klinische und serologisch-experimentelle Untersuchungen. Verlag Hans Huber, Bern, Stuttgart.

6. Hoigné, R. and Däppen, U. (1963) Schweiz. Rundsch. Med. Prax. 52, Nr. 3, 61-67.

7. Hoigné, R., Keller, H., Sonntag, R. (1988a) Penicillins, cephalosporins and tetracyclines; In: Meyler's Side Effects of Drugs. Chapter 26 (Chief Editor M.N.G. Dukes), Elsevier Science Publishers B.V., Amsterdam, New York, Oxford, pp. 501-542.

8. Hoigné, R., Maurer, P., Wymann, R., Müller, U., Hess, T., Jordi, A., Maibach, R. (1988b) Häufigkeit von Arzneimittelexanthemen. Meeting of the Deutsche Dermatologie-Gesellschaft; Proceedings of the 35th Congress, 27 Apr-1 May, Munich, F.R.G. (O. Braun-Falco and S. Borelli Eds), Hautarzt (in press).

9. Hoigné, R., Sonntag, M.R., Zoppi, M., Hess, T., Maibach, R., Fritschy, D. (1987) New Engl. J. Med. 16, No. 19, 1217.

10. Hoigné, R., Stocker, F., Middleton, P. (1983) Epidemiology of drug allergy; Drug monitoring. Handbook of Experimental Pharmacology, Vol. 63 (A.L. de Weck and H. Bundguard, Eds), Springer-Verlag Berlin, Heidelberg, pp. 187-205.

11. Idsøe, O., Guthe, T., Willcox, R.R., and de Weck, A.L. (1969) Schweiz. med. Wschr. 99, 1190-1197, 1221-1229, 1252-1257.

12. Mayer, R.L. (1933) Toxicodermien, Hb. Haut- und Geschlechtskrankheiten, Vol. IV/2, Springer, Berlin, p. 1.

13. Neftel, K.A., Hauser, S.P., Müller, M.R. (1985) J. Infect. Dis. 52, 90-98.

R. Hoigné et al.

14. Neftel, K.A. and Hübscher, U. (1987) Antimicrob. Agents Chemother. 31, No. 11, 1657-1661.

15. von Pirquet, C. und Schick, B. (1905) Die Serumkrankheit. Deutike Verlag, Leipzig/Wien.

16. Westerman, G., Corman, A., Stelos, P., Nodine, J.H. (1966) J.A.M.A. 198, 193-194.

AAS 29:
Risk Factors for
Adverse Drug Reactions
© 1990 Birkhäuser Verlag Basel

DRUG DEVELOPMENT OPTIMIZATION - BENZODIAZEPINES

M. Lader

Abstract

The benzodiazepines are among the most widely-used of drugs. Sedative effects are common but tend to lessen after a few days, although cognitive effects may persist. Car accidents and falls in the elderly are the most serious practical consequences. On discontinuation, a variety of syndromes are encountered, including relapse, rebound, and withdrawal. Anxiety disorders tend to be remitting and relapsing rather than chronic. Withdrawal follows a characteristic course and symptom pattern, perceptual hypersensitivity being common and distressing. The syndrome is worse after stopping shorter-acting than longer-acting benzodiazepines.

Benzodiazepines are prescribed for many different mental and physical conditions, sometimes inappropriately. Chronic use for twelve months or more ranges from 0.5% of the adult population in Sweden through 1.8% in the U.S.A., 3.1% in the U.K., and 6.8% in Belgium.

Benzodiazepines differ with respect to elimination half-life and potency. High-potency compounds may be particularly likely to induce sedation, memory disturbance and perhaps dependence. Partial agonists may be less of a problem in these respects. Newer compounds include benzodiazepines with selectivity on one or other of the putative subclasses of receptor, partial inverse agonists and antagonists, compounds acting near the benzodiazepine complex, and new drugs, such as buspirone, believed to act primarily on 5-HT pathways.

M. H. Lader

Introduction

The benzodiazepines are among the most widely-used of drugs. However, in many countries their popularity is waning as prescribers become more aware of problems with unwanted effects and with rebound and withdrawal syndromes. The earlier benzodiazepines were long-acting, and it was thought that their shorter-acting successors would have important advantages. Other developments include partial agonists and partial inverse agonists, compounds acting on the benzodiazepine-GABA macro-molecular site although not as a typical benzodiazepine, and anxiolytic agents acting on 5-HT pathways directly. I shall review the problems of unwanted effects and dependence, mainly from an epidemiological view-point, and then relate the pharmacological properties of the newer com-pounds to possible differences in their clinical profile of adverse effects.

Adverse behavioural effects

Benzodiazepines are used, inter alia, as anxiolytics and hyp-notics. The latter use exploits the sedative actions which occur at higher than anxiolytic doses. The sedation should disappear by the time the patient wakes up. Hypnotics are thus unique in that their wanted effect and unwanted effect are identical - sedation - but separated in time by about 8 hours.

The sedative effects are well known and the subjective feel-ings of tiredness generally show tolerance within a few days. Psycho-motor performance can be markedly affected, especially in normal sub-jects (Wittenborn, 1979), and cognitive and memory functioning may be impaired (Hendler et al., 1980; Curran, 1986). Many such studies involve single-dose administration in normal subjects, and on repeated dosage tolerance tends to occur (Lader et al., 1980), although the EEG changes and some memory defects may not show tolerance. Interference with psychological functioning is more difficult to show in patients (Bond et al., 1974a) because anxiety itself impairs functioning (Bond et al., 1974b), and lessening that anxiety may result in improved psychological functioning.

These adverse effects can have practical social consequences such as impaired car-driving. Many studies have attempted to evaluate the possible contribution of benzodiazepines to road accidents. These have included laboratory-based studies of simulated car-driving behaviour, experimental studies of actual car-driving, and epidemiological surveys among subjects involved in accidents (Bauer, 1984; Landauer, 1981). Benzodiazepines affect simulated driving such as increasing reaction times and speed of driving. Actual driving performance, either on a test course or in real traffic conditions, is impaired by tranquillizers but the effects are often inconsistent. Moreover, the relevance of such studies to the effects in anxious patients is not clearly established.

Epidemiological studies suffer from the problems of recruiting an appropriate control group and also from the difficulty of establishing the effects of anxiety itself on driving ability. Consequently, no clear findings have emerged although several studies (e.g. Binnie, 1983) suggest a statistically increased risk of having an accident in benzodiazepine users compared with controls. Notwithstanding, the contribution of benzodiazepines to traffic accidents is trivial compared with the heavy toll induced by alcohol. The interaction of benzodiazepines with alcohol is particularly hazardous (Seppala et al., 1979).

One type of accident over-represented in benzodiazepine users is falls in the elderly. Kramer and Schoen (1984), in the U.S.A., found that 70% of patients over 70 years of age who had fallen over had been taking the long-acting hypnotic, flurazepam, compared with 19% of those not falling over. Dizziness, fainting, blackout, and falls are commoner in the elderly taking tranquillizers than in the drug-free (Hale et al., 1985).

Dependence on benzodiazepines

When these drugs were introduced in the early 1960's, it was already known that physical dependence supervened after long-term high-dose usage as evidenced by a major withdrawal syndrome including fits and delirium (Hollister et al., 1961). Under other conditions of usage the risk of dependence was deemed low, certainly much lower than that associated with barbiturates (Marks, 1978). Although much dispute continues concerning both the nature and frequency of the syndromes seen after discontinuation of benzodiazepines, almost everyone acknowledges that they are common. The main controversy is whether the symptoms represent relapse, the gradual return of the original symptoms; rebound where the symptoms are initially more severe than pre-treatment but subside rapidly; or withdrawal comprising new symptoms which sometimes persist for weeks or even months.

A recent study throws doubt on the chronic nature of many anxiety disorders (Rickels et al., 1988). Anxious patients stopping clorazepate, a long-acting benzodiazepine, experienced rebound and withdrawal, whereas those stopping buspirone, a non-benzodiazepine tranquillizer, did not. Nor did those stopping buspirone show significant relapse, suggesting that many anxiety disorders remit and perhaps later relapse, rather than remaining at chronically high anxiety levels indefinitely.

Rebound and withdrawal are contiguous or even overlapping syndromes. Rebound was described for hypnotic benzodiazepines (Kales et al., 1978), and rebound anxiety was subsequently noted following the anxiolytic benzodiazepines, especially in patients discontinuing shorter-acting benzodiazepines such as lorazepam, alprazolam, and bromazepam (Fontaine et al., 1984; Pecknold et al., 1988). Rebound occurs in many patients stopping a benzodiazepine even after only short-term use, especially in those taking higher doses. Although the syndrome is usually mild and subsides within a few days, the anxiety, tension and insomnia may be distressing and result in resumption of the drug.

Withdrawal is characterized by a cluster of symptoms occurring at a time after discontinuation related to the elimination half-life of the drug. Its features include anxiety, insomnia and tension together with depression, lack of energy, depersonalization, headache, nausea, tremor and loss of appetite. Perceptual symptoms include hyperacusis and hyperosmia, sore eyes and photophobia, hypersensitivity to touch and pain and to bright light. Experience of motion, misperceptions and paranoid ideas have also been recorded. About 20-40% of long-term normal dose users experience a withdrawal syndrome, which in a few can be severe and prolonged (Ashton, 1984). As with rebound, shorter-acting compounds are associated with prompt, severe withdrawal syndromes which the patient attributes to stopping the drug (Tyrer et al., 1981; Busto et al., 1986). It is not known whether such compounds <u>induce</u> dependence more frequently than do longer-acting compounds.

The likelihood, but perhaps not the severity, of withdrawal phenomena increases with dose (Hallstrom and Lader, 1981). Duration of usage might seem to be crucial and indeed several studies show that the incidence of withdrawal is greater after long-term than short-term use (e.g. Rickels et al., 1983). As rebound can come on quite quickly in short-term use, it may be rather that the rebound-prone subject experiences difficulties and subsequently goes on to long-term use because he cannot discontinue.

The abuse potential of benzodiazepines is generally low, but they are increasingly used by polydrug abusers to cushion withdrawal from opioids. More ominously, intravenous use of temazepam has become apparent in the U.K., where liquid-filled capsules are available and primary benzodiazepine addiction is an increasing problem.

Extent of usage

A broader perspective of the epidemiological implications of benzodiazepine use is available from estimates of usage, particularly in term of number of users. Patterns of use differ among countries, reflecting different health-care delivery systems, varying diagnostic practices and even differing dosage regimens. In the last respect the "defined daily dose" (DDD) system is helpful (Lunde et al., 1979). Problems also arise in trying to translate consumption figures into numbers of users and finally in trying to assess whether such usage is appropriate and justified.

Across countries, the overall average exposure to tranquillizers in the industrialized countries ranges from 1-3 "standard units" (one week of therapy) per head of adult population, the higher figures pertaining to France and Belgium, the U.S.A. and U.K. being around 1.2. The leading benzodiazepines world-wide are diazepam, lorazepam, and alprazolam. However, sales figures cannot be used as evidence of inappropriate use, of possible abuse or dependence, or as a basis for social concern about adverse effects.

Most prescriptions for benzodiazepines represent continuing therapy for chronic problems. The proportion of repeat to total prescriptions for tranquillizers in the U.K. has risen in the past 20 years from less than a quarter to over three quarters (Marks, 1983). Presumably few newly presenting patients are placed on benzodiazepines but despite that a cohort of chronic users has accrued. About a half of those given prescriptions for benzodiazepine tranquillizers have a primary diagnosis of a mental disorder, the rest being for a wide range of somatic disorders (Williams, 1978), especially circulatory, digestive and musculoskeletal problems, as well as even more ill-defined conditions (Mulvihill et al., 1985). About a third of the patients who received a tranquillizer were judged appropriately treated; 12% of those not given a tranquillizer were judged to need one.

Surveys of use by representative samples of the general population rely on the accuracy of the information elicited from the interviewee. A study in 1971 found the 1-year prevalence of tranquillizer use to range between 9.7% and 16.8% of the adult population across the various countries surveyed (Balter et al., 1974). A study 10 years later revealed a slightly wider range of prevalence of users (7.4-17.6%), but with some overall fall off in use (Balter et al., 1984). Across all countries, usage was higher in females than males; in females, peak usage was in the 45-65 age range, in males it was more uniform across ages. Chronic use, i.e. for at least the previous 12 months, ranged from 0.5% of the adult population in Sweden to 5.8% in Belgium, the figures for the U.S. A. and the U.K. being 1.8 and 3.1%, respectively. As a percentage of all users, these figures translate into 14.2% and 27.4% in the U.S.A. and U.K. It is hardly surprising that public concern in the U.K. is greater than that in the U.S.A.

A survey of long-term use in the U.S.A. showed such users to be mainly older and female, with high levels of emotional distress and chronic somatic health problems (Mellinger et al., 1984). Most were monitored by a physician.

The development of long-term use was studied by Williams et al. (1982) in a prospective longitudinal survey. About one fifth of patients given a psychotropic drug continued on that medication beyond six months. The factors most predictive of long-term use were age over 45, previous use of psychotropic drugs, severity of psychiatric disorder and chronic social problems (Murray et al., 1982). Many patients lacked social support, and they attributed the onset of their symptoms to a life crisis.

Differences among benzodiazepines

Against this background we can now evaluate the various ways in which new compounds have been and are being developed. The first step was the synthesis and evaluation of shorter-acting benzodiazepines to complement the earliest benzodiazepines which were all long-acting and/ or had long-acting metabolites (e.g. chlordiazepoxide, diazepam, nitrazepam, and flurazepam). The main examples are oxazepam, lorazepam and alprazolam among those marketed as anxiolytics, temazepam and triazolam among the hypnotics.

A large number of studies have evaluated the sedative actions of the different types of benzodiazepines. It has clearly emerged, in line with prediction from pharmacokinetic data, that the shorter-acting hypnotics are associated with little if any sedation the next morning, in contrast to the long-acting compounds which persist the next day after a single dose and accumulate on repeated administration. With day-time anxiolytics, sedation after shorter-acting compounds is usually transitory but may persist in the susceptible. Dosage is an important factor: after high doses of a short-acting hypnotic, residual effects may be easily detected the next day.

The relative lack of residual effects with shorter-acting hypnotics is counterbalanced by greater problems on discontinuation. Even after short-term use, rebound - that is, an increase in insomnia beyond pre-treatment levels - may be a problem. Triazolam, which is very short-acting, is more troublesome than temazepam and lormetazepam, especially in higher dose (0.5 mg and above) (Lader & Lawson, 1987). The danger with rebound is that the patient recommences his medication and develops tolerance and dependence. With day-time use as well, rebound anxiety may follow discontinuation, and again shorter-acting compounds like lorazepam are associated with more rebound than longer-acting drugs.

These clinical differences are predictable to a large extent from the pharmacokinetic properties of the individual benzodiazepines.

However, various lines of evidence suggest some pharmacodynamic differences with some benzodiazepines presenting particular problems. In general, high-potency compounds are associated with more clinical reports of sedation, psychomotor, cognitive and memory impairment and paradoxical effects than are the lower-potency compounds. In addition, dependence problems are regarded as worse with drugs like lorazepam and alprazolam. By contrast, oxazepam, a low-potency, shorter-acting compound, is not usually associated with a severe withdrawal syndrome.

We have directly compared lorazepam and oxazepam in single doses given to normal subjects with respect to a range of measures (Curran et al., 1987). On psychomotor and subjective variables 15 mg of oxazepam was equivalent equivalent to 1 mg of lorazepam, and 30 mg of oxazepam and 2 mg of lorazepam had about double the effect. However, on some memory variables, the 2-mg dose had a disproportionately great effect. Similarly, in a laboratory paradigm of the release of hostility, 2 mg of lorazepam was particularly powerful (Bond & Lader, 1988).

Using an analogy from the opioid field, one might speculate that the low-potency benzodiazepines are partial agonists whereas the high-potency compounds are full agonists. This difference is not important with respect to anxiolytic, hypnotic, and muscle-relaxant therapeutic effects nor for subjective sedative or psychomotor effects. However, memory impairment, release of aggression, rebound, and dependence are worse with the full than the partial agonists. I emphasize this is only a working hypothesis.

Newer compounds

The discovery of specific high-affinity binding sites for benzodiazepines 10 years ago has led to important research culminating in the amino acid sequencing of the $GABA_A$-benzodiazepine-chloride ionophore macromolecule. Despite this, the identity, and even the existence, of the naturally occurring ligand remains obscure. Subdivisions of the receptor types into "central" and "peripheral" is well established, although it is now apparent that the latter receptors are also found in the brain. The possible division of the central receptors into "Type I" and "Type II" subtypes is, however, still controversial. Most benzodiazepines do not distinguish between the two types, which may indeed reflect differences in the membrane environment rather than distinct subtypes (Lo & Snyder, 1983). Claims that compounds selective for Type I receptors might be anxiolytic without sedation remain to be investigated. The lack of a putative selective Type II ligand hampers research in this area. In particular, it is unclear whether the Type II receptors are linked to GABA mechanisms or not.

One fascinating and so far unique aspect of benzodiazepine neuropharmacology is the existence of three kinds of ligands - benzodiazepine-like agonists, which increase GABA function and inhibit neuronal activity; inverse agonists which decrease GABA function and excite neurons, causing convulsions and anxiety; antagonists which block the actions of both types of agonist. The existence of inverse agonists reflects the presence in the complex of two allosterically linked receptors (Ehlert, 1986). In practical terms, a range of compounds can be envisaged, ranging from full agonists at one end through partial agonists, antagonists and partial inverse agonists to full inverse agonists. An important clinical question is whether partial agonists might be anxiolytic without being sedative, and several such compounds are presently under evaluation. Partial inverse agonists are being studied as potential agents in the treatment of cognitive deficit states such as the dementias.

Other compounds developed as anxiolytics and hypnotics act on or near the benzodiazepine complex. These drugs include alpidem and zuriclone as anxiolytics, zolpidem and zopiclone as hypnotics. In general, these compounds have less propensity to produce side effects than do clinically equivalent doses of typical benzodiazepines but their dependence potential is still being evaluated.

Finally, an interesting portfolio of anxiolytics and putative anxiolytics has developed containing compounds acting on various 5-HT receptor subtypes. They include $5-HT_{1A}$ agonists such as buspirone, gepirone and ipsapirone, $5-HT_2$ antagonists like ritanserin and $5-HT_3$ antagonists like zacopride. Of these only buspirone is in clinical use; it produces little if any sedation, and discontinuation does not seem so far to be associated with rebound or withdrawal phenomena. However, the onset of action is rather slow, and nausea and headache can be troublesome side effects.

M. H. Lader

References

1. Ashton, H. (1984) Br. Med. J. 288, 1135-40.

2. Balter, M.B., Levine, J., and Manheimer, D.I. (1974) New Eng. J. Med. 290, 769-774.

3. Balter, M.B., Manheimer, D.I., Mellinger, D.G., and Uhlenhuth, E.H. (1984) Curr. Med. Res. Opin. 8, (suppl. 4), 5-18.

4. Bauer, R.L. (1984) Public Health Report 99, 573-574.

5. Binnie, G.A.C. (1983) Br. Med. J. 287, 1349-1350.

6. Bond, A.J., James, D.C., and Lader, M.H. (1974a) Psychol. Med. 4, 374-380.

7. Bond, A.J., James, D.C., and Lader, M.H. (1974b) Psychol. Med. 4, 364-373.

8. Bond, A.J., and Lader, M. (1988) Psychopharmacol. 95, 369-373.

9. Busto, U., Sellers, E.M., Naranjo, C.A., Cappell, H., Sanchez-Craig, C.M., and Sykora, K. (1986) New Eng. J. Med. 315, 854-859.

10. Corda, M.G., Giorgi, O., Longoni, B., Ongini, E., Barnett, A., Montaldo, S., and Biggio, G. (1988) J. Neurochem. 50, 681-687.

11. Curran, V.H. (1986) Biol. Psychol. 23, 179-213.

12. Curran, H.V., Schiwy, W., and Lader, M. (1987) Psychopharmacol. 92, 358-364.

13. Ehlert, F.J. (1986) Trends Pharmacol. Sci. 7, 28-32.

14. Fontaine, R., Chouinard, G., and Annable, L. (1984) Am. J. Psychiatry 141, 848-852.

15. Hale, W.E., Stewart, R.B., and Marks, R.G. (1985) Drug Intell. Clin. Pharm. 19, 37-40.

16. Hallstrom, C., and Lader, M. (1981) Int. Pharmacopsychiat. 16, 235-244.

17. Hendler, N., Cimini, C., Terence, M.A., and Long, D. (1980) Am. J. Psychiatry 137, 828-30.

18. Hollister, L.E., Motzenbecker, F.P., and Degan, R.O. (1961) Psychopharmacologia 2, 63-68.

19. Kales, A., Scharf, M.B., and Kales, J.D. (1978) Science 201, 1039-1041.

20. Kramer, M., and Schoen, L.S. (1984) J. Clin. Psychiatry 45, 176-177.

21. Lader, M.H., Curry, S., and Baker, W.J. (1980) Br. J. Clin. Pharmacol. 9, 83-90.

22. Lader, M.H., and Lawson, C. (1987) Clin. Neuropharmacol. 10, 291-312.

23. Landauer, A.A. (1981) Br. Med. J. Aust. 1, 624-626.

24. Lo, M.M.S., and Snyder, S.H. (1983) J. Neurosci. 3, 2270-2279.

25. Lunde, P.K.M., Baksaas, I., Halse, M., Halvorsen, I.K., Stromnes, B., and Oydvin, K. (1979) In: Studies in Drug Utilization (U. Bergman, A. Grimsson, A.H.W. Wahba and B. Westerholm, Eds), WHO Regional Publications, European Series 8, Copenhagen, pp. 17-28.

26. Marks, J. (1978) "The Benzodiazepines. Use, overuse, misuse and abuse". MTP Press, Lancaster.

27. Marks, J. (1983) Neuropsychobiol. 10, 115-126.

28. Mellinger, G.D., Balter, M.B., and Uhlenhuth, E.H. (1984) J. Am. Med. Assoc. 251, 375-379.

29. Mulvihill, M.N., Suljaga, P.K., Falkenstein, J., and Ehr, A.P. (1985) Mt. Sinai J. Med. 52, 276-280.

30. Murray, J., Williams, P., and Clare, A. (1982) Soc. Sci. Med. 16, 1595-1598.

31. Pecknold, J.C., Swinson, R.P., Kuch, K., Lewis, C.P. (1988) Arch. Gen. Psychiatry 45, 429-436.

32. Rickels, K.L., Case, W.G., Downing, R.W., and Winokur, A. (1983) J. Am. Med. Assoc. 250, 767-771.

33. Rickels, K., Schweizer, E., Csanalsoi, I., and Case, G. (1988) Arch. Gen. Psychiatry 45, 444-450.

34. Seppala, T., Linnoila, M., and Mattila, M.J. (1979) Drugs 17, 389-401.

35. Tyrer, P., Rutherford, D., and Huggett, T. (1981) Lancet 1, 520-522.

36. Williams, P. (1978) Psychol. Med. 8, 683-693.

37. Williams, P., Murray, J., and Clare, A. (1982) Psychol. Med. 12, 201-206.

38. Wittenborn, J.R. (1979) Br. J. Clin. Pharmacol. 7, 61S-76S.

AAS 29:
Risk Factors for
Adverse Drug Reactions
© 1990 Birkhäuser Verlag Basel

EXTRAPYRAMIDAL SYMPTOMS
IN NEUROLEPTIC RECIPIENTS

R. Grohmann, R. Koch and L.G. Schmidt

Abstract

Adverse drug reactions (ADRs) in psychiatric therapy were continously assessed in the AMÜP study (AMÜP = Arzneimittelüberwachung in der Psychiatrie (drug surveillance in psychiatry)) conducted at two psychiatric university departments in the F.R.G. The Intensive Drug Monitoring (IDM) method was used to monitor 1107 patients, 754 of whom received neuroleptics (NLs). As is the rule in clinical psychiatric practice, polypharmacy was frequent, with combinations of two neuroleptics and combinations of a neuroleptic and an antiparkinson drug ranking first and second, respectively.

Extrapyramidal motor symptoms (EPMS) were observed in 35% of the NL patients. In most cases they required a change in medication, usually addition of an antiparkinson drug. In about one quarter of all EPMS cases, withdrawal of the imputed NL was necessary. Parkinsonism was the most frequent single symptom, followed by acute dystonia and akathisia. Differences in EPMS rates between the two most frequently used neuroleptics, haloperidol, a high-potency butyrophenone, and perazine, a medium-potency phenothiazine, were distinct. EPMS were observed with haloperidol in 56% and attributed to haloperidol alone in 92% of these cases. With perazine, an EMPS occurred at a rate of only 14%, and in 37% of the cases EMPS were attributable to perazine in combination with other NLs. Age, sex, diagnosis and dosage of administered NLs were closely interrelated. For instance, NL patients over 60 years of age were almost exclusively female, the majority of them being endogenous depressives, whereas in younger patients the diagnosis of schizophrenia prevailed. Therefore, analysis of potential risk factors for development of EPMS must simultaneously include diagnosis, sex and age as well as concomitant physical disease, duration and dosage of all drugs administered before development of EPMS. However, the small case numbers in some subgroups, as we found them in this study based on everyday clinical practice, will probably be a limiting factor in such multivariate analyses.

Introduction

Extrapyramidal motor symptoms (EPMS) are well-known adverse effects of neuroleptic drugs. Four different types of EPMS are distinguished: **1. acute dystonia,** a tonic contraction - preferentially of the orofacial muscles - which results in forced tongue excursions, opening of the mouth, torticollis or oculogyric crisis as most typical manifestations; as a rule it occurs during the first days of treatment; **2. parkinsonism,** characterized by muscular rigidity and hypokinesia; tremor may be present as well, and more rarely there is only tremor; **3. akathisia,** a state of driven restlessness in which the patient feels unable to sit or lie still; parkinsonism and akathisia occur for days to weeks after initiation of neuroleptic treatment; **4. tardive dyskinesia,** involuntary movements most commonly of bucco-linguo-masticatory muscles resulting in facial grimacing, lip-smacking, chewing movements or writhing excursions of the tongue. It usually develops only after months or years of neuroleptic therapy.

Parkinsonism was immediately described as a side effect of neuroleptic drugs when they were first used as antipsychotics (Delay & Deniker, 1952), and the recognition of acute dystonia and akathisia - and some years later also of tardive dyskinesia - as adverse effects of neuroleptics followed (Steck, 1954; Kulenkampff & Tarnow, 1956; Uhrbrand & Faurbye, 1960). A large number of papers has been published on the subject of EPMS since that time; however incidence figures vary greatly, and as regards the occurrence of EPMS under the conditions of everyday clinical practice, the results from Ayd's (1961) survey of 3,775 inpatients treated with neuroleptics are still the most frequently cited ones. He described the frequencies and types of EPMS onnected with various neuroleptics in use at the time and recognized age and sex as potential risk factors. Many new drugs have been marketed in the meantime, but with the exception of clozapine all of them induce EPMS symptoms similar to the early antipsychotic agents; the relative weight of potential risk factors for occurrence of EPMS in individual patients remains unclear. But in contrast to internal medicine, where drug surveillance programmes like the Boston Collaborative Drug Surveillance Study (Jick, 1970) have been established on a large scale since the midsixties in order to satisfy the need for epidemiological data on frequencies and types of adverse drug reactions (ADRs) for early detection of new effects and identification of potential risk factors, no such study was undertaken in psychiatry for a long time.

In order to fill this need, the AMÜP study (AMÜP = Arzneimittelüberwachung in der Psychiatrie (drug surveillance in psychiatry)) was initiated by the German neuropharmacological and pharmacopsychiatric association, the Arbeitsgemeinschaft für Neuropsychopharmakologie und Pharmakopsychiatrie (AGNP), in 1979. The aim of the study was to assess ADRs in psychiatric inpatients under the conditions of everyday clinical practice. With the financial support of the German Federal Health Office, the Bundesgesundheitsamt, the AMÜP study has been in progress for ten years now. This paper presents the data from the AMÜP study which concern EPMS in neuroleptic recipients.

Definitions and Methods

The psychiatric departments of the Free University of Berlin and of the University of Munich collaborated in the AMÜP study for the entire period of data collection (May 1979 to December 1986). For the purposes of this study, the following definitions were used.

Adverse drug reaction (ADR) was defined as meaning any drug-related manifestation in a patient which was unintended and undesired by the prescribing physician. Symptoms due to intoxication and inefficacy were not classified as ADRs (Seidl et al., 1965).

Probability of a causal relationship between an unwanted manifestation and treatment (Seidl et al., 1965; Hurwitz & Wade, 1969) was rated

> **possible**, if the ADR was not characteristic of the drug in question, and/or the sequence of events was not in agreement with previous experience;
>
> **probable**, if the adverse reaction to the drug in question was generally accepted
>
> - and the sequence of events was in agreement with previous experience
> - and the probability of an alternative cause was less than 50%;
>
> **definite**, if, in addition to the criteria required for classification of an ADR as "probable", recurrence of the ADR necessarily followed rechallenge with the drug(s) in question.

Severity of ADR was implicitly determined by rating the ADR's impact on therapy as follows.

> **Grade I**; the ADR did not lead to any change in medication.
>
> **Grade II**; the ADR led to a change in medication in the form of dose reduction and/or additional treatment to counteract the ADR.
>
> **Grade III**; the ADR led to the discontinuation of the medication suspected of causing the ADR (including cases in which the drug would have been discontinued, had it not been vital).
>
> In addition, it was decided on clinical grounds whether an ADR was to be considered severe or even life-threatening.

Inpatient surveillance involved two different methods:

1. intensive drug monitoring (IDM), in which a randomly selected sample of patients (approx. 150 per year) was monitored for all ADRs throughout their stay in hospital during May 1979-December 1986 period; and

2. organized spontaneous reporting (OSR), which assessed only grade-III ADRs in all other inpatients at the participating hospitals.

Drug use per year was continously assessed for the calculation of relative risk rates.

More detailed descriptions of our methodological approach have previously been published along with first results (Rüther et al., 1980; Grohmann et al., 1984; Schmidt et al., 1984).

The present paper reports the results as obtained by IDM and OSR at the Psychiatric Departments of the Free University of Berlin and the University of Munich, covering the time from May 1979 to December 1986. If not explicitly stated otherwise, the ADRs included in this paper were all "probable" or "definite".

Results

With IDM, a total of 1,107 inpatients were monitored, 754 of whom received neuroleptics (NLs). Polypharmacy was common practice in these patients. Haloperidol and perazine, the two most frequently used NLs, were combined for at least one day in 111 patients, which corresponds to 28% and 33% of the haloperidol and perazine patients, respectively. Haloperidol was also frequently combined with levomepromazine (38% of the haloperidol patients), biperiden (51%), benzodiazepines (37%) or tricyclic antidepressants (28%). The high rate of polypharmacy led to the imputation of drug combinations in ADRs in a number of cases, where drugs with similar ADR profiles were combined and additive effects suspected. Therefore, ADR rates for single drugs or drug groups are given as rates for all cases as well as for cases, in which the drug in question was imputed alone (single drug imputation (s.d.i.)).

EPMS rates

EPMS were observed in 34.7% of all NL patients; only in 16 cases (2.1%) were other drug groups - lithium salts and antidepressants (mostly in cases of tremor) - involved in EMPS, in combination with NLs. EPMS required a change in medication in 84% of cases; discontinuation of the NL was necessary in about one quarter of EPMS cases, or 8.1% of all NL patients. As shown in Table 1, there is a great difference in EPMS rates between the high-potency and the medium/low-potency NLs as groups as well as between the most frequently used representatives of these

R. Grohmann et al.

groups, haloperidol and perazine or levomepromazine. In addition, the ratio of s.d.i. to all cases was smaller in medium-potency NLs (63% with perazine) in comparison with high-potency haloperidol, which was mostly imputed alone (in 92%) in EPMS. The lower EPMS rates found even in high-potency **depot** preparations reflect that, as a rule, they are used in a later phase of treatment, when patients who have been stabilized on oral medication are switched to a depot before dismissal.

Table 1: EPMS in neuroleptic (NL) recipients. Rates for groups and sub-groups of drugs, and for single drugs (IDM, probable/definite cases).

	No. of patients	All grades	All s.d.i.*	All grade II/III	All grade III
All neuroleptics	754	34.7	32.6	29.3	8.1
High-potency NLs	476	51.1	46.8	43.5	12.0
Medium-potency NLs	551	11.8	7.1	8.3	1.9
Low-potency NLs	94	0	0	0	0
Haloperidol	395	55.9	51.6	48.6	12.7
Fluspirilene	71	16.9	7.0	15.5	4.2
Flupentixol-D	32	12.5	9.4	12.5	3.1
Perazine	340	14.4	9.1	9.7	2.1
Levomepromazine	255	5.1	0.8	4.3	0.4
Thioridazine	102	6.9	5.9	4.9	1.0
Clozapine	54	0	0	0	0

* single drug imputation

Types of EPMS

As shown in Table 2, parkinsonism was the most frequent extra-pyramidal motor symptom in all the NL as well as the haloperidol patients, followed by acute dystonia and akathisia. In the university hospital population under study, tardive dyskinesia developing as a new ADR in the course of the investigation period was observed in only 1.3% of all NL patients. Haloperidol, used in 52.3% of the NL patients, was involved in 87.3% of all cases of parkinsonism, and in 88.6%, 78.6% and 70% of all cases of acute dystonia, akathisia and tardive dyskinesia, respectively .

Table 2: Types of extrapyramidal motor syndrom (EPMS) with all neuroleptics and with haloperidol (IDM, probable/definite cases).

	Percentage of NL patients (n=754)		
	All grades	Grade II/III	Grade III
Parkinsonism	17.1	13.8	4.4
Acute dystonia	13.9	12.9	1.1
Akathisia	11.1	9.4	3.3
Tardive dyskinesia	1.3	0.9	0.8

	Percentage of haloperidol patients (n=395)		
	All grades	Grade II/III	Grade III
Parkinsonism	28.6	23.1	7.9
Acute dystonia	23.5	22.0	1.5
Akathisia	16.7	14.4	5.3
Tardive dyskinesia	2.5	1.3	1.0

As regards the **time of onset,** 75% of the acute cases of halo-peridol-induced dystonia became manifest within the first eight days of treatment, while 75% of the cases of parkinsonism and akathisia were observed within the first 18 and 21 days of treatment, respectively.

Differences in EPMS rates according to diagnosis

With haloperidol, distinctly different EPMS rates were found in different diagnostic groups. In the schizophrenia group (which also included paranoid states), 60.9% of 225 haloperidol patients experienced EPMS of grade II/III. Manic patients (n=22) came second with an EPMS rate of 45.4%. In other diagnostic groups (endogenous depression, n=99; organic psychiatric disorders, n=25, and neurosis, n=16), the EPMS rate was 31-32%. These differences were paralleled by differences in the average daily dose of haloperidol: 17.5 mg/day in the schizophrenia group, 16.0 mg/day in manic patients and 8.1-10.0 mg/day in the other three groups.

Age, sex and **diagnosis** were closely interrelated, as can be seen from Table 3; most of the younger patients suffered from schizo-phrenia, whereas most of the patients over 60 years of age had a diag-nosis of endogenous depression, the majority of them being female. This subdivision of the data resulted in very small case numbers for some age and sex groups.

Even in the much larger population monitored by OSR (2,957 haloperidol patients in the schizophrenia group and 708 endogenous depressives exposed to haloperidol), only 18 males and 47 females were under the age of 30 and only 64 males over 60 years of age in the depression group; as few as 13 males were over 60 in the schizophrenia group. Therefore, in this population, too, evaluation of ADR rates related to age, sex and diagnosis is hampered by small numbers of cases.

Severe EPMS

Neuroleptic malignant syndrome (NMS), the most severe and potentially lethal EPMS complication, which is characterized by severe muscular rigidity, stupor or coma, hyperthermia and autonomic dysfunc-tion, was observed as a probable ADR in two cases, and in one case NMS was suspected ('possible' case). In both of the probable cases halo-peridol was involved, once on its own and once in combination with penfluridol and levomepromazine, which corresponds to an all-cases rate of 0.04% in all 5,229 patients exposed to haloperidol or of 0.02% in all 10,445 patients exposed to any neuroleptic drug.

Another severe type of EPMS, the neuroleptic syndrome characterized by severe parkinsonism and stupor, but without vegetative signs, was observed as a probable ADR in 8 NL patients (0.08%), 7 of whom had received haloperidol (0.13%) and one trifluperidol. In 4 patients parkinsonism was accompanied by severe depression with suicidal ideation as a probable ADR to NLs; haloperidol was imputed twice.

Table 3: Numbers of patients exposed to haloperidol, broken down accord-ing to age, sex and diagnosis (IDM).

Age	Sex	Total numbers	Schizophrenia group	Endogenous depression group	Others
<30	m	59	47	4	8
	f	63	46	9	8
<60	m	81	43	15	23
	f	131	78	31	22
>60	m	9	3	5	1
	f	52	8	35	9
All	m	149	93	24	32
All	f	246	132	75	39
All	m+f	395	225	99	71

Discussion

The overall EPMS frequency of 35% found in neuroleptic recipients in the AMÜP study is similar to that observed in earlier surveys.
Ayd (1961) and Ananth (1971) found EPMS in 39% and 33% of NL recipients,
respectively. With regard to parkinsonism, our result (17%) is in excellent agreement with Ayd's figure (15%), but obvious differences exist
with respect to akathisia and acute dystonia (21% and 2% in Ayd's population versus 11% and 14% in our study, respectively). However, Ayd did
not state his method of assessment, and in contrast to our study, patients with several EPMS symptoms were classified only for one symptom.
Finally, his patients were all on phenothiazines, whereas in this study
butyrophenones prevail among the high-potency NLs. Swett (1975) observed
acute dystonia in 10.1% of all patients, in 9% of the phenothiazine
patients and in 16% of the haloperidol patients, which is similar to our
findings. Moleman et al. (1982) retrospectively examined EPMS in 98
haloperidol patients. They observed an overall EPMS rate of 55% and
parkinsonism, akathisia and dystonia rates of 38%, 23% and 12%, respectively. These figures are in fairly good agreement with our results in
haloperidol patients, with the exception of acute dystonia, which was
seen twice as often in our IDM patients. As Moleman et al. did not state
the frequencies of the diagnoses in their patients and gave only their
average age, these factors may be responsible for the difference in the
rate of acute dystonia. Moleman and associates found a correlation
between higher dose and higher frequency of parkinsonism. The higher
medium daily dose probably also accounts for the higher rate of EPMS in
schizophrenic patients observed in this study in comparison with depres-
sive patients. The relative frequency of tardive dyskinesia in our
study, 1.3%, underestimates its true incidence, as in this university
hospital population acutely ill patients predominate; chronic patients
with a history of long-term NL treatment prevail in the state hospitals.
When these patients are included, the estimated frequency of tardive
dyskinesia is 15-20% (Gerlach & Casey, 1988).

As regards the time of onset, the more protracted appearance
of acute dystonia in this study (75% in the first week) differs markedly
from the data reported by Ayd, who observed 90% of acute dystonia cases
within the first three days of NL treatment. Possibly, the frequent use

of levomepromazine in addition to haloperidol during the very first days of treatment offers an explanation, since in a number of cases the acute dystonia appears after discontinuation of levomepromazine. This finding is evidence in favour of a protective effect of this type of combination, though more detailed analysis is still necessary.

Neuroleptic malignant syndrome, the most severe EPMS, was observed to have a lower incidence (0.02% in 10,445 NL patients) than has been reported in the literature so far. Keck (1987) observed NMS in 0.9% of 679 patients, and Guze and Baxter (1985) arrived at an estimate of 0.5-1.0%. The figure reported by Gelenberg et al. (1988) comes closest to ours, their NMS rate being 0.07% in 1,470 NL patients. As it is well established that the incidence rates of rare events, such as NMS, can be reliably assessed only after monitoring large samples of patients (Stephens, 1985), differences in sample size probably account for the lower rate observed in our study.

In summary, the data on EPMS from the AMÜP study presented above show that such an epidemiological study produces reliable results for the relative frequency of various ADRs, even for rare events, on account of the large sample size at our disposal after 8 years of data collection. In addition, the methodological approach chosen for IDM allows us to assess the observed ADRs' clinical relevance by rating their impact on therapy.

Analysis of age and sex distribution in different diagnostic groups shows that these factors are closely interrelated and in turn relate to drug dosage and comedication. Therefore, univariate, one-by-one analysis of these factors does not lead to meaningful results. Multivariate analyses are necessary and will soon be published. However, they may have severe limitations due to the inhomogeneous distribution of patients, which results in very small case numbers for some subgroups - as demonstrated above in the case of haloperidol. Yet this is what we encounter under the actual conditions of everyday clinical practice at university psychiatric departments.

References

1. Ananth, J.V., Ban, T.A., Lehmann, H.D., Rizvi, F.A. (1971) Amer. J. Psychiat. 127, 75-80.

2. Ayd, F.J. (1961) J.A.M.A. 175, 1054-1060.

3. Delay,J., Deniker, P. (1952) In: Pharmako-Psychiatrie (Selbach, H., Eds.), Darmstadt, Wissenschaftliche Buchgemeinschaft, pp. 85-9.

4. Gelenberg,A.J., Bellinghausen, B., Wojcik, J.D., Falk, W.E., Sachs, G.S. (1988) Amer. J. Psychiat. 145, 517-518.

5. Gerlach, J., Casey, D.E. (1988) Acta psychiat. scand. 77, 369-378.

6. Grohmann,R., Hippius, H., Müller-Oerlinghausen, B., Rüther, E., Scherer, J., Schmidt, L.G., Strauss, A., Wolf, B. (1984) Eur. J. Clin. Pharm. 26, 727-734.

7. Guze, B.H., Baxter, L.R. (1985) New Engl. J. Med. 313, 163-166.

8. Hurwitz, N., Wade, O.L. (1969) Br. Med. J. 1, 531-536.

9. Jick, H., Miettinen, O.S., Shapiro, S., Lewis, G.P., Siskind, V., Slone, D. (1970) J.A.M.A. 213, 1455-1460.

10. Keck,P.E. jr., Pope, H.G. jr., Mc Elroy, S.L. (1987) Amer. J. Psychiat. 144, 1344-1346.

11. Kulenkampff, C., Tarnow, G. (1956) Nervenarzt 27, 178-181.

12. Moleman, P., Schmitz, P.J.M., Ladee, G.A. (1982) J. Clin. Psychiat. 43, 492-496.

13. Rüther, E., Benkert, O., Eckmann, F., Eckmann, I., Grohmann, R., Helmchen, H., Hippius, H., Müller-Oerlinghausen, B., Poser, W., Schmidt, L., Stille, G., Strauss, A., Überla, K. (1980) Arznei-mittel-Forsch./Drug Res. 30, 1181-1183.

14. Schmidt,L.G., Grohmann, R., Helmchen, H., Langscheid-Schmidt, K., Müller-Oerlinghausen, B., Poser, W., Rüther, E., Scherer, J., Strauss, A., Wolf, B. (1984) Acta psychiatr. scand. 70, 77-89.

15. Steck, H. (1954) Ann. Medicopsychol. 112, 734-743.

16. Stephens, M.D.B. (1985) Stockton Press, New York, pp. 9-13.

17. Swett, C. (1975) Amer. J. Psychiat. 132, 532-534.

18. Uhrbrand, L., Faurbye, A. (1960) Psychopharmacologia 1, 408-418.

19. Seidl,L.G., Thornton, G.F., Cluff, L.D. (1965) Am. J. Public Health 55, 1170-1175.

AAS 29:
Risk Factors for
Adverse Drug Reactions
© 1990 Birkhäuser Verlag Basel

EPIDEMIOLOGICAL SCREENING
FOR POTENTIALLY CARCINOGENIC DRUGS

G. D. Friedman and J. V. Selby

Abstract

This paper describes a unique program for the systematic screening of commonly used prescription drugs for possible carcinogenic effects, by following up a large cohort of patients with computer-stored pharmacy data for incidence of cancer. Among the most interesting findings in recent analyses are an association of several antibiotics with subsequent lung cancer, and negative associations of prescribed vitamin E and diazepam with certain cancers. Analyses of additional data do not clearly indicate that these represent causal relationships to the drugs themselves. Also of interest is our continuing negative evidence regarding reserpine and metronidazol. The planned computerization of all pharmacies in our medical care program, now serving over 2.2 million subscribers, should greatly increase our drug surveillance capabilities.

Introductory remark

We have engaged in what some investigators derisively call a "fishing expedition". We would like to describe this fishing expedition and some of the things that we have learned from it.

G. D. Friedman and J. V. Selby

Origins of our drug-cancer surveillance study

The program started when our department, the Division of Research (formerly, Department of Medical Methods Research), Kaiser Permanente Medical Care Program, Northern California Region, received a contract from the U.S. Food and Drug Administration to develop and implement a pilot Drug Reaction Monitoring System in one of our medical care centers, our San Francisco facility. The Kaiser Permanente Medical Care Program is a large health maintenance organization that provides comprehensive medical care, both outpatient and inpatient, to its subscribers on a prepaid basis. About one quarter of the persons living in the San Francisco Bay Area and other parts of Northern California are members; the total number served in the region is now about 2.2 million. This subscriber population is quite heterogeneous, both ethnically and socioeconomically (Hiatt & Friedman, 1982).

Under the Drug Reaction Monitoring System a computer-based data entry system was developed for all outpatient prescriptions issued from the pharmacies in the San Francisco facility, which then served a subscriber population numbering about 120,000 persons at any one time. When the FDA contract ended in mid-1970, other support permitted pharmacy data collection to proceed until mid-1973. Thus, between July 1969 and August 1973, a total of 1,307,767 prescriptions for 3,446 drug products dispensed to 149,139 patients were recorded.

Because each subscriber is issued a unique medical record number that is recorded at all visits to the program, these pharmacy data could be readily linked to clinical event data. Our initial data analyses focused on the incidence of various outpatient diagnoses in users as compared with nonusers of various drugs. For example, we could clearly demonstrate a strong association between the use of oral contraceptives and the short-term incidence of vaginal candidiasis (Friedman et al., 1971). We also found that the majority of outpatient prescriptions dispensed were for a relatively small number of drugs (Friedman, 1972). We were faced then, as we are now, with the plethora of statistical associations that fishing expeditions generate; thus we had to give considerable thought to the meaning of these associations and how to select those that were more apt to lead to meaningful findings (Friedman, 1972).

In the mid-1970s, the National Cancer Institute requested applications for grants to study drugs as possible predisposing factors for cancer. It seemed to us that our unique computer-stored pharmacy data and our ability to link these records to subsequent cancer occurrence provided an excellent opportunity for such a study. The fear that drugs might be causally linked to cancer was heightened by a few well-known carcinogenic drugs and by the fact that drugs are ingested in considerably larger doses than other environmental chemicals of concern. Fortunately, we were awarded a grant and were able to proceed with the study.

Methods

We defined our study cohort as the 143,574 persons in the data base with sufficient identifying information that they could be classified as to age and sex. Follow-up for cancer employed two main sources of data. One was the program's computer-stored file of all hospitalizations in the region. The other was the SEER (Surveillance, Epidemiology, and End Results) program registry of all cancer cases in the San Francisco Bay Area, now operated by the Northern California Cancer Center. Due to errors uncovered by our early analyses we soon decided to review the medical records of every case obtained from these data sources. The resulting set of cancer cases, verified as to both diagnosis and date of diagnosis, has been very valuable for other epidemiologic studies as well as the drug studies.

Cohort members are followed up for cancer development for as long as they remain subscribers to the program. With the help of the California Resource for Cancer Epidemiology we performed a validation study on about 10,000 subjects, searching for cancers listed from other sources but not recorded in our data. The small number of cases absent from our records had little effect on the sensitivity of our screening analyses (see below) (Friedman, in press). Thus we are satisfied with our present follow-up system.

In our biennial screening analyses we study the incidence of cancer among users of each of 215 (then) commonly used drugs. We tabulate the observed and expected numbers of cases of cancer at each site, all lymphomas and leukemias combined, and all sites combined. The expected numbers are based on the age-sex-specific incidence of cancers in the entire study cohort. Keeping in mind the limitations of hypothesis-seeking analyses of this kind, we note statistically significant excesses and deficits of observed cases. We also allow for lag periods in follow-up in an attempt to rule out artifactual drug-cancer associations due to the prescription of the drug for early symptoms of the cancer (Friedman & Ury, 1980).

The associations resulting from this screening process are considered as potential hypotheses for further study. Some can be readily dismissed as likely the result of confounding. For example, an association of bronchodilator drugs with subsequent lung cancer is most likely due to the use of these drugs for pulmonary conditions caused by cigarette smoking, which is also the main cause of lung cancer. Others call for further, more detailed investigation. This involves obtaining additional data by manual review of medical records, or by exploring additional computer-stored data sources such as information collected from some of the patients during multiphasic health checkups. Limits to the availability of personnel have led to two approaches to medical record review. For a few very promising or otherwise important hypotheses we perform full case-control studies requiring the review of hundreds of medical records. For associations that seem less likely to be due to a drug effect, we perform quick reviews -- usually of only the cases of cancer among users of the drug of interest and an equal number of users who did not develop the cancer. This gives us a "feel" for whether there is confounding by indication for the drug, whether there is a dose-response relationship, and whether chance or other factors seem likely explanations for the association.

Results of our latest screening analyses

We have conducted our screening analyses on biennial updates of cancer follow-up since 1976. Our latest results through 1984, presented in detail elsewhere (Selby & Friedman, submitted), will illustrate what this fishing expedition produces.

In screening 215 drugs against cancers at 56 sites, there were 227 statistically significant ($p < 0.05$, two-tailed) associations: 170 positive and 57 negative. The numbers expected purely by chance (not simply 5% of the total, in light of complex statistical considerations beyond the scope of this paper) were 120 positive and 30 negative associations (Selby & Friedman, submitted). Thus, the larger observed number very likely includes some nonchance associations, due to either confounding factors or real drug effects.

An example of a drug with positive associations that are likely due to a confounding factor is folic acid (Table 1). This vitamin has turned up with positive associations ever since we first studied it in 1978. Some of the excess cancers are those known to be alcohol- or tobacco-related. Since folic acid is often prescribed for anemia or presumed nutritional deficiencies connected with heavy consumption of alcohol, it is easy to see why it would appear linked to alcohol-related

Table 1: Statistically significant ($p < 0.05$) associations with folic acid. Follow-up through 1984; 248 users.

| Cancer site | Number of cases | | SMR[+] |
	Observed	Expected	
Oropharynx	2	0.08	26.0**
Hypopharynx	2	0.04	46.5***
Bladder	3	0.52	5.8*
Myeloid leukemia	2	0.14	14.1*
All cancer	30	11.52	2.6***

[+] SMR: Standardized morbidity ratio

* $p < 0.05$

** $p < 0.01$

*** $p < 0.002$

cancers. The small-scale chart review confirmed that a diagnosis of alcoholism was often found in the medical records of folic acid recipients (Friedman & Ury, 1983).

Another drug with some interesting positive associations was the antibiotic, erythromycin (Table 2). Review of the charts of the 14 erythromycin users who developed multiple myeloma did not reveal differences in duration or intensity of erythromycin use as compared to 28 randomly selected age- and sex-matched erythromycin users who did not develop the condition. Nor were obvious confounding factors suggested by the indications for erythromycin use. In the absence of better evidence for a causal or confounded relationship, it is likely that this is merely a chance association.

In contrast with the specific relationship of multiple myeloma to just one antibiotic, erythromycin, lung cancer risk was increased among users of ampicillin, tetracycline, cephalexin, cloxacillin, and sulfamethoxazole, as well as erythromycin. At first glance this appeared to be an artefact; either the antibiotics were given for pulmonary infections secondary to the presence of lung cancer, or for pulmonary or other infections secondary to cigarette smoking, which in turn caused

Table 2: Statistically significant associations with erythromycin and results for all cancer. Follow-up through 1984; 13,941 users.

| Cancer site | Number of cases | | SMR[+] |
	Observed	Expected	
Lung	86	59.5	1.4***
Multiple myeloma	14	5.1	2.7***
All cancer	454	425.8	1.1

[+] SMR: Standardized morbidity ratio

*** p<0.002

the lung cancer. The first possibility was ruled out by our lag analyses. The associations persisted for cancers diagnosed more than two years after the antibiotics were prescribed. The second was ruled out when we noted in the outpatient diagnosis file, created at the time of the prescription file, that the antibiotics were prescribed as often for nonsmoking-related as for smoking-related conditions. Also, among 30,567 pharmacy users who had computer-stored multiphasic checkup data, the association was not reduced when smoking habits were taken into account. Thus, the associations appear to be real, but since a diverse group of drugs was involved, our hypothesis is that susceptibility to infection rather than the drugs themselves, may be associated with a heightened susceptibility to lung cancer.

Some of the negative associations were also intriguing. A possible protective effect was shown for prescribed vitamin E in relation to all cancers combined. This was strongest in the follow-up data through 1982 (Table 3). Because dietary vitamin E has been considered as a possible preventive factor for cancer, we investigated this association further. The deficit of cancer cases was present almost exclusively in women, and the sites most affected were breast, lung, and colon. The

Table 3: Negative association of prescribed vitamin E with all cancer and findings for breast, colon, and lung cancer. Follow-up through 1982; 436 users.

Cancer site	Number of cases		SMR+
	Observed	Expected	
All cancer	23	34.5	0.7*
Breast	1	4.7	0.2
Colon	3	4.5	0.7
Lung	3	5.2	0.6

+ SMR: Standardized morbidity ratio

* $p < 0.05$

strongest negative relationship was present in persons who received only one prescription for vitamin E; thus there was no apparent dose-response effect. Further exploration revealed that 85.6% of the prescriptions came from the otolaryngology clinic, and almost all of these from one physician. The main indications for prescription -- tinnitus, vertigo, and sensorineural hearing loss -- were not themselves associated with a reduced risk of cancer. All in all, we were not convinced that a protective effect of prescribed vitamin E was demonstrated. The reason for the reduced incidence of cancer in this small group of women is elusive; this may well be just a chance finding.

Negative associations were also observed for the anxiolytic drug, diazepam, with two forms of malignancy, colon cancer and Hodgkin's disease (Table 4). Because of the concern raised that diazepam use may lead to breast cancer it was also reassuring to note the similarity between observed and expected cases for this site.

Table 4: Statistically significant associations (negative) with diazepam and findings for breast cancer and all cancer. Follow-up through 1984; 12,928 users.

| Cancer site | Number of cases | | SMR[+] |
	Observed	Expected	
Colon	57	79.9	0.7**
Hodgkin's	0	4.7	0.0*
Breast	155	143.8	1.1
All cancer	807	784.0	1.0

+ SMR: Standardized morbidity ratio

* $p < 0.05$

** $p < 0.01$

Absent associations

As for diazepam and breast cancer, this study has provided valuable negative evidence in that we have found no associations for several drugs implicated in other studies in humans or animals.

One example is reserpine, which was suspected of increasing risk for breast cancer in early epidemiologic studies. Most later studies did not confirm this relationship (International Agency for Research on Cancer, 1987). In an attempt to reconcile divergent findings, Williams et al. hypothesized that reserpine increased risk only for breast cancer occurring after age 50 and only in women who used the drug for at least 5 years (Williams et al., 1978). We found no relationship of reserpine and breast cancer overall in our data, but conducted additional analyses to test Williams' hypothesis directly (Friedman, 1983a). We could not confirm it.

Other valuable negative results came from our analyses of metronidazol, which was found to increase the incidence of tumors of the lung and lymphoma in rats and tumors of the breast, colon, liver, pituitary gland, and testis in mice. As did the Mayo Clinic group (Beard et al., 1988), we found little in our follow-up studies of humans to support the animal data (Friedman & Selby, 1989). An increased risk of cancer of the uterine cervix in our data was probably due to common risk factors for both vaginal trichomoniasis (which is treated with metronidazol) and cervical cancer, or to increased detection of cervical cancer in patients with vaginitis.

Barbiturates and lung cancer

Probably our most interesting positive finding to date is an association between barbiturate use and lung cancer. This showed up in our first analyses of follow-up data through 1976 (Friedman, 1981). Users of three barbiturates, pentobarbital, phenobarbital, and secobarbital all showed increased risk of lung cancer (Table 5) and these associations persisted in the lag analysis, which ignored cases diagnosed during the first two years after the drug was dispensed. Since cigarette smokers tended to use barbiturates more often than nonsmokers, we performed further analyses of subjects who had multiphasic health checkups. The barbiturate-lung cancer association was present among smokers, exsmokers, and nonsmokers. Unfortunately, the data for non-smokers, the most critical group for demonstrating the independence of a barbiturate effect on lung cancer risk, was unreliable due to small numbers of cases - four observed and 2.7 expected.

Computer-stored data suggested a dose response effect. A low-dose barbiturate mixture of phenobarbital and belladonna showed a slightly raised standardized morbidity ratio (observed/expected cases) of 1.2, intermediate between that of users of the above barbiturates and nonusers. Moreover, the standardized morbidity ratio rose from 1.7 for all barbiturate users to 2.9 for persons who received at least two prescriptions of barbiturates to 4.8 for persons who received at least three (Friedman, 1983).

We also conducted chart review studies to compare: 1) lung cancer cases with and without computer-recorded barbiturate use, and 2) barbiturate users who did and did not develop lung cancer. Barbiturate-

Table 5: Findings for barbiturates and lung cancer. Follow-up through 1976. Data from Friedman & Ury (1983).

Drug	Number of users	Number of users		SMR[+]
		Observed	Expected	
Pentobarbital	2,156	34	12.3	2.8***
Phenobarbital	5,834	44	28.9	1.5*
Secobarbital	2,884	27	15.0	1.8**
Any of above	9,816	87	50.2	1.7***

[+] SMR: Standardized morbidity ratio

* $p < 0.05$

** $p < 0.01$

*** $p < 0.002$

associated lung cancer cases did not differ significantly from other cases with respect to histological type or location of the tumor. Barbiturate users who developed lung cancer did not differ significantly from other barbiturate users with respect to duration or frequency of barbiturate use. Thus, the chart review data did not support a causal association.

Causality is biologically plausible since barbiturates can induce enzymes which convert potential carcinogens into their active forms. Also, phenobarbital has been shown to promote the growth of tumors in experimental animals.

In our latest follow-up data through 1984, pentobarbital continues to show statistically significant positive associations with cancers of the lung (51 observed and 24.1 expected cases, $p < 0.002$), thyroid (6 observed, 1.4 expected cases, $p < 0.01$), and all sites combined (212 observed, 167.2 expected cases, $p < 0.002$). Secobarbital was associated with cancer of the small bowel (4 observed, 0.7 expected cases, $p < 0.01$). Phenobarbital now shows positive associations with cancer of the gallbladder (8 observed, 3.2 expected cases, $p < 0.05$) and bone (3 observed, 0.6 expected cases, $p < 0.05$), and negative associations with cancers of the colon (36 observed, 50.1 expected cases, $p < 0.05$) and bladder (8 observed, 18.0 expected cases, $p < 0.05$). The association of lung cancer with the latter two barbiturates is smaller than before and no longer statistically significant. The reduction or disappearance of a definite positive association after longer follow-up does not rule out a causal effect. It may indicate that the effect is short-term promotion of tumor growth rather than long-latency initiation.

We cannot conclude from our data that barbiturates are carcinogenic in humans. We have therefore begun a larger case-control study of lung cancer in which the complete medical records of 250 lung cancer cases and 400 controls are reviewed and compared for a history of barbiturate exposure. Cases and controls have been carefully matched on cigarette smoking history to control for this likely confounder. The study includes 50 cases of lung cancer in persons who never smoked (with four controls per case).

G. D. Friedman and J. V. Selby

Significance of this project

To our knowledge this is the only systematic program of screening of large numbers of medicinal drugs for carcinogenic effects, by means of a prospective cohort study. The International Agency for Research on Cancer (IARC) evaluated the carcinogenic effects of 48 drugs and drug groups by 1987 (IARC, 1987). We have published data on 15 of these drugs. Our findings were cited by IARC for ten of these drugs, and our studies were the IARC's only source of human data for three - phenazopyridine, sulfisoxazole, and sulfamethoxazole.

In view of the many positive associations that we observe in our screening analyses and the likelihood that few if any represent true drug effects, we have approached the dissemination of our findings very cautiously to avoid alarming the public unnecessarily. We have published our screening findings in specialized cancer journals with emphasis on the fact that the associations observed should only be viewed as hypotheses for further study.

We view the associations in our data not only as clues to drug carcinogenesis but also as clues to other cancer-causing factors for which a drug might be a marker. Thus in evaluating phenylbutazone by case-control study (Friedman, 1982), we concluded that an association with leukemia was probably due to the latter's association with musculo-skeletal disease for which the drug was used. Similarly, as noted above, our working hypothesis for the antibiotic-lung cancer association is that susceptibility to infection underlies the relationship.

We believe that one of the most important results of our work to date is the negative findings that have been observed for drugs about which suspicion has been raised, either from laboratory data or from other epidemiologic studies. This reassurance must be tempered by two caveats. One is the limited statistical power to detect associations for all but the most commonly used drugs. The second is the limited duration (11 to 15 years) of follow-up to date, which may not reveal carcinogenic effects with longer latency.

With these reservations, our overall impression based on results of the study to date is that commonly prescribed medicinal drugs used in the course of ordinary clinical care, other than the well-known exceptions such as postmenopausal estrogens and cancer chemotherapeutic drugs, are not a significant cause of cancer.

Future plans

Continued analysis of the 1969-1973 pharmacy cohort is still important. We are beginning now to get into the two-decade latency interval that may reveal the initiating phase of carcinogenesis. Many of the drugs dispensed at that time are still commonly used. We recently listed the 50 drugs most commonly dispensed to the program's outpatients and found 36 of them in the 1969-1973 pharmacy data (Friedman, in press).

Yet there are many important and commonly used drugs that were introduced after 1973. These include several nonsteroidal anti-inflammatory agents, beta-blockers, calcium channel blockers, histamine H_2 receptor antagonists, and new cardiac, antihypertensive and psychoactive drugs. We would like to perform similar studies on these.

We have collected data from several hundred thousand prescriptions dispensed in the 1980s (Friedman, in press) and can use these as a basis for forming new cohorts. More promising still is our program's plan to connect all of its pharmacies to a central computer system. Implementation is occurring in phases across our 14 medical centers, from 1989 through 1991, at which time we will have a data collection system that enables us to link drug use for over 2,200,000 subscribers to subsequent adverse events, including the development of cancer.

It is evident that we plan to continue and expand our fishing expedition. Our experience suggests that fishing is not a bad thing to do, if 1) when one catches a fish, it is carefully and properly prepared before serving, and 2) one recognizes that not catching fish while fishing can also be rewarding.

Acknowledgment

Our work was supported by grants R37 CA19939 and R35 CA49761 from the National Cancer Institute.

G. D. Friedman and J. V. Selby

References

1. Beard, C.N., Noller, K.L., O'Fallon, W.M., et al. (1988) Mayo Clin. Proc. 63, 147-153.

2. Friedman, G.D. (1972) J. Chronic Dis. 25, 11-20.

3. Friedman, G.D. (1981) J. Natl. Cancer Inst. 67, 291-295.

4. Friedman, G.D. (1982) J. Chronic Dis. 35, 233-243.

5. Friedman, G.D. (1983) Int. J. Epidemiol. 12, 375-376.

6. Friedman, G.D. (1983a) J. Chronic Dis. 36, 367-370.

7. Friedman, G.D. (In press) In: Pharmacoepidemiology: The Science of Postmarketing Drug Surveillance (B.L. Strom, Ed), Churchill Livingstone, New York.

8. Friedman, G.D., and Selby, J.V. (1989) J. Am. Med. Assoc. 261, 866.

9. Friedman, G.D., and Ury, H.K. (1980) J. Natl. Cancer Inst. 65, 723-733.

10. Friedman, G.D., and Ury, H.K. (1983) J. Natl. Cancer Inst. 71, 1165-1175.

11. Friedman, G.D., Collen, M.F., Harris, L.E., Van Brunt, E.E., and Davis, L.S. (1971) J. Am. Med. Assoc. 217, 567-572.

12. Hiatt, R.A., and Friedman, G.D. (1982) Kidney Int. 22, 63-68.

13. International Agency for Research on Cancer. (1987) In: IARC Monographs on the evaluation of the carcinogenic risk of chemicals to humans (Suppl 7), vol. 1-42. IARC, Lyon, France.

14. Selby, J.V., and Friedman, G.D. (Submitted) Screening prescription drugs for possible carcinogenicity: eleven to fifteen years of follow-up.

15. Williams, R.R., Feinleib, M., Connor, R.J., and Stegens, N.L. (1978) J. Natl. Cancer Inst. 61, 327-335.

SHORT COMMUNICATIONS

AAS 29:
Risk Factors for
Adverse Drug Reactions
© 1990 Birkhäuser Verlag Basel

MONITORING FOR ADVERSE PREGNANCY OUTCOMES
RELATED TO DRUG EXPOSURE DURING PREGNANCY

E. Andrews and P. Tennis

Although there has been concern over increased risk of birth
defects from drug exposure during pregnancy ever since the thalidomide
scare, the actual measurement of increased risk of birth defects is
often difficult to accomplish. Methodological issues include the deter-
mination of the exact timing of exposure, definition of outcome, knowledge of other risk factors, and sample size considerations. Such studies
often require relatively large sample sizes because outcomes expected
and drug exposures during pregnancy are relatively rare and because the
magnitude of increased risk related to the drug exposure is often not
very large.

We have developed an overall strategy for monitoring pregnancies exposed to acyclovir. This strategy includes a prospective registry
of exposed pregnancies, a case-control study, prescription event monitoring study, and a follow-up study to determine whether genital herpes,
the condition for which acyclovir is used, produced increased risk. This
follow-up study, which is to be be published elsewhere in full detail at
a later stage, involves record linkage of data from a US health maintenance organization. Also, it is important to discuss the strengths and
weaknesses of each methodology.

AAS 29:
Risk Factors for
Adverse Drug Reactions
© 1990 Birkhäuser Verlag Basel

A TWENTY-YEAR FOLLOW-UP STUDY ON PHENACETIN ABUSE

U.C. Dubach

The study

The rate of analgesic drug abuse in Switzerland is estimated at 0.005-0.2%, with a preponderance in certain regions, notably the Basle area and the northwestern part of the country (where there is chemical industry and watch manufacturing). In Basle, the number of dialysis patients with analgesic nephropathy reached an all-time high of 40% in 1981. Due to the importance of the problem we began a prospective epidemiological study in 1968 on 623 working women, aged 30-49 years, regularly taking tablets containing phenacetin. The control group of 621 female nonusers were matched for age, maritial status, parity, nationality and type of work. Phenacetin consumption was assessed and checked by urine tests.

Results

Morbidity

After 11 years of follow-up with yearly checks, specific gravity of urine following thirst was lower by 23.3.% in the group of abusers versus 6.7% in the controls. Serum creatinine was elevated in 6.7% of the abusers versus 0.9% of the controls. No difference was observed as regards the occurrence of bacteriuria, proteinuria or haematuria. Therefore, the occurrence of renal damage, as reflected by the serum creatinine levels, was about 10 times higher in the group of analgesic abusers and 6 times higher in the same population with impaired urinary concentration ability of the kidney after quenching thirst.

Mortality

The mortality results were completed after 20 years (1968-1987) on 89% of the original cohort, since out of 1,247 women, 101 died during the study period and 135 were lost to follow-up. With respect to overall mortality, the relative risk in the study group was 2.2 versus the controls. However, renal and urogenital causes of death, when analysed separately by means of life table analysis revealed a markedly increased relative risk of 16.1 versus controls. The risk is positively correlated with the amount of phenacetin ingested over time. Results on cardiovascular and tumour mortality after 20 years of follow-up will be reported elsewhere in detail.

No excess risk could be demonstrated with respect to salicylate use.

References

1. Dubach, U.C., Levy, P.S., Rosner, B., et al. (1975) Lancet I, 539-43.

2. Dubach, U.C., Rosner, B., and Pfister, E. (1983) New Engl. Med. J. 308, 357-62.

AAS 29:
Risk Factors for
Adverse Drug Reactions
© 1990 Birkhäuser Verlag Basel

PHYSICIAN'S COMPLIANCE

The term "compliance" refers to discipline on the part of the patient and means his or her acting according to rules and health professionals' instructions. The latter are lacking in 50-80% of all patients treated for hypertension, though it is still the patients, and not the physicians, who are primarily considered to be non-compliant. Our observations in the management of hypertensive outpatients, however, have revealed that the lack of compliance is rather more on the part of the physicians.

The management of hypertension is a process which, for therapy to be successful, requires several steps spanning from the first observation of increased blood pressure (BP) to the optimization of treatment. Investigations as to the quality of antihypertensive therapy reveal shortcomings on all levels of this complicated process. The aim of a study carried out at the outpatients' department of the Medizinische Universitäts-Poliklinik in Basle was to define both the type and the extent of such shortcomings in therapy.

In the first phase of our investigations, the present state, or initial situation, was defined, revealing a 53%-dropout rate at the level of the first measurement of increased BP and a 54%-patient dropout at the level of the institution of indicated therapy. Our residents were confronted with these unsatisfactory results, instructed according to the guidelines published by the Swiss Society Against High Blood Pressure and lectured on important international publications on this topic.

U.C. Dubach

Phase two followed. Again, patient dropout rates of 57% and 48% were observed. In the third phase, increased BP was recorded on a punch card by a nurse, and patients were recalled by letter. By means of this simple administrative procedure we succeeded in reducing dropout rates from 50% down to 30% at the level of the first registration of increased BP, and from 50% down to 17% in the treatment phase.

Conclusion

The introduction of nonmedical staff and administrative meas-ures (punch card registry) into therapy leads to a significant reduction in dropout rates and to an improvement of physician's compliance.

References

1. Conen, D., Berner, U., and Dubach, U.C. (1982) Schweiz. med. Schr. 112, 1925-1927.

2. Conen, D. (1984) In: Die Qualität ärztlicher Leistungen. Eine Evaluation des diagnostischen und therapeutischen Prozesses, Verlag Hans Huber, Berne, Stuttgart, Vienna, pp. 72-90.

AAS 29:
Risk Factors for
Adverse Drug Reactions
© 1990 Birkhäuser Verlag Basel

COMPLIANCE WITH SHORT-TERM
HIGH-DOSE ETHINYL OESTRADIOL IN YOUNG PATIENTS
WITH PRIMARY INFERTILITY

New Insights from the Use of Electronic Devices

W. Kruse, W. Eggert-Kruse, J. Rampmaier, B. Runnebaum and E. Weber

Abstract

The objective of the study was to investigate patient compliance with ethinyl oestradiol therapy. Medication was prescribed to be taken in 20-µg doses four times daily for seven days. Oestrogens are prescribed for standardization of the cervical mucus before the sperm cervical-mucus penetration test (SCMPT) is performed. Relation of drug compliance with adverse drug reactions reported by the patients.

The methodology used in this study was continual microprocessor-based monitoring by means of the Medication Event Monitoring System, MEMS ^{TM}. Adverse drug reactions were recorded by means of standardized interviews.

Investigations were carried out on thirty female patients, mean age: 28.8 years (range 21 to 36 years), with primary infertility, mean duration of infertility: 3.9 years (range 9 months to 8 years).

The results showed that individual patients' compliance was remarkably variable, ranging from 14.3% up to 136%. The average compliance was 65%. Less than 30% of the prescribed doses were taken on schedule. Administration of oestrogens was effective in all but one patient. High cervical indices were documented irrespectively of the dose taken. In answer to the questionnaire, 24 out of 30 women reported side effects, of which 79% were rated by the patients as being mild. The lower the drug compliance was, the more adverse reactions were reported. In patients who took more than 65% of the drug, this inverse relationship was statistically significant ($r = -0.71$, $p = <0.01$).

Our conclusion is that the empirically fixed daily dose of 80 µg of ethinyl oestradiol for seven days appeared to be too high in regard of the observed dose response, i.e. cervical mucus quality. A dose finding study, including compliance monitoring, seems to be reasonable. Within further studies, a simpler dosage regimen should also be taken into account. The observed association between patients' reports of adverse effects and drug compliance deserves further investigation.

Introduction

There are numerous reasons why patients deviate from prescribed drug regimens. Although it is generally assumed that adverse drug reactions (ADRs) may influence drug compliance, available information concerning this aspect of compliance is sparse (Haynes, 1979). In studies in which patients have been asked for their reasons for non-compliance, side effects were infrequently mentioned. However, in a placebo-controlled study with two anti-inflammatory drugs, compliant patients reported fewer subjective side effects than less compliant patients (Joyce, 1962). The difference was statistically significant for both drugs, and for placebo too. Therefore, it seemed promising to study the possible relationship between ADRs and compliance.

Patients and methods

Compliance with high-dose ethinyl oestradiol was monitored in female patients with primary infertility attending the infertility unit of the University Women's Hospital. The mean age of the women was 28.8 years with a range of 21 to 36 years. The mean duration of infertility was 3.9 years with a range of 9 months to 8 years.

Since 1985 the sperm-cervical mucus penetration test (SCMPT) has been an established part of the diagnostic investigations in infertile couples. It has been proven as a reliable predictor of pregnancy (Eggert-Kruse et al., 1989). Because of hormonal standardization of the cervical mucus quality, 80 µg of ethinlyoestradiol were administered daily for 7 days before the SCMPT was performed. The cervical index was assigned according to several criteria (Insler et al., 1972). Microprocessor-based monitors (Medication Event Monitoring System, MEMS[TM], APREX Corp. Fremont, Calif., U.S.A.) were used for compliance assessment. Continuous compliance monitoring has been shown to be practicable in ambulatory patients on long-term treatment. It allowed correlation with clinical events (Kruse & Weber, in press; Kruse, 1988). An accuracy of 100% has been demonstrated for the measurement of interdose intervals by microelectronic monitoring in comparison with a standard laboratory clock (Rudd et al., 1981). Continuous compliance monitoring has the potential to elucidate the relationship between dose and response (Kruse, 1989).

The MEMS[TM] bottles were standard U.S. pill bottles, each fitted with a childproof cap that contained a microprocessor. Each opening and closing of the bottle was recorded as a presumptive dose. Data were retrieved by connecting the medication container to a microcomputer communication port. Compliance data were obtained as listings of the date and time of individual bottle openings and closings, the duration of opening, and the hours since the previous dose. From the time pattern of openings information is yielded about patients' adherence to the prescribed QID regimen. Compliance was expressed quantitatively; it was defined as: number of doses taken during period divided by the number of prescribed doses during period multiplied by 100 and expressed in percent.

The SCMPT, the purpose of drug intake and the dosage regimen were explained to the patients as usual during their first visit to the clinic. They were provided with the medication filled into the monitors and told to return the medication container when attending the clinic for the SCMPT. Patients were not informed about the compliance monitoring. Between the first visit and the beginning of drug intake there was an average time interval of 11 days. The drug was usually administered from the 7th to 14th day of the menstrual cycle. During the second visit the SCMPT was carried out, and the patients were interviewed about drug adverse effects which they might have experienced. The interview begun with an open question, which was followed by questions from a standardized questionnaire (Spriet & Simon, 1985). All patients were interviewed by the same investigator. The patients were asked to rate symptoms related to ADRs as mild, moderate or severe. The design of the study is shown in Figure 1.

Descriptive statistical evaluation was performed by means of Student's t-test and Pearson Correlation Coefficients using a computer package program (SAS). Data are presented as means ±SD, median values and ranges.

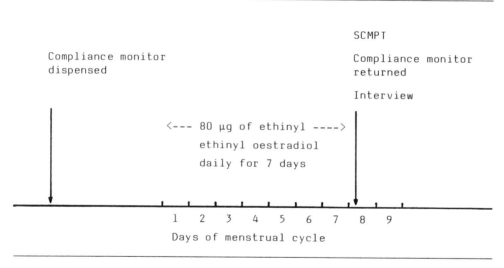

Figure 1: Design of the study.

Results

Thirty-five patients were randomly selected. Five patients had to be excluded from the study, two of which became pregnant and did not use the drug. In the third case, data retrieval from the monitor was defect. The remaining two patients failed to return the monitor despite the fact that they were contacted by mail.

The monitoring revealed a remarkable variability in individual compliance in the remaining 30 patients, ranging from 14.3% to 136% (Table 1). The average compliance was 65%. Patients' adherence to the prescribed QID regimen was poor. Less than 30% of the prescribed doses were taken on schedule, corresponding to two days out of the seven. The study population could be separated into two groups on account of the compliance rates. Fifteen patients out of 30 complied with the seven-day course of drug intake whereas another 15 failed to take the drug for seven days exactly (Table 2). Drug intake either began too late or was stopped too early, or vice versa. A patient-initiated drug holiday was recognized in one patient. Patients who took the drug for less than seven days did not adhere to the QID regimen either. This behaviour was also reflected by the average dosing interval, which was as twice as long than in compliant patients (6.9 h vs. 13.3 h).

Table 1: Compliance with 20 µg of ethinyl oestradiol QID for seven days in 30 young patients with primary infertility.

	range	mean+SD	median	28 tablets prescribed
Compliance (intake, % of prescribed doses)	14.3–136	64.9+30.9	65	18 tablets taken (mean)
Period covered by drug intake (days)	3 – 10	6.5+ 1.5	7	
Period covered by drug intake on QID schedule (days)	0 – 8	2.0+ 2.4	2	
Adherence to prescribed regimen (% of doses taken on QID schedule)	0 –114	34.3+35.6	28.6	8 tablets taken on schedule (mean)

Table 2: Adherence to prescribed QID regimen (80 µg of ethinyl oestradiol daily) in 30 patients.

Patients		15	12	3
Duration of drug intake (days)		7	<7	>7
% of prescribed doses taken	Median	82.1	30.3	103.0
	Range	50 -110.7	14.3- 78.6	67.9-136
Days covered by drug intake on schedule	Median	2	0	5
	Range	0 - 7	0 - 3	2 - 8
% of doses taken on schedule	Median	43	0	62.5
	Range	0 -100	0 - 42.8	28.5-114
Dosing interval (hours)	Median	6.9	13.3	6.3
	Range	5.0- 11.8	5.5- 42.2	5.6- 12.2

Administration of oestrogens was effective in all but one patient. Except for one, all samples of cervical mucus were of high quality, and the median cervical index was 11 (range 9-12). High indices were documented irrespective of the dose of ethinyl oestradiol taken. The one exception was due to local alterations after conisation.

ADRs were reported spontaneously or in answer to an open question by 16 patients out of 30. Twenty-four women reported side effects in answer to the standardized questionnaire. Six patients did not complain of side effects at all. The symptoms reported are listed in Tables 3 and 4. Seventy-nine percent of symptoms were rated by patients as being mild. The frequency of symptoms reported as severe was comparable with the 4% recorded by physicians in a previous study (Eggert-Kruse et al., 1989). All symptoms reported are well known to be possibly related to the intake of oestrogens (Murad & Haynes, 1980).

The lower drug compliance was, the more adverse reactions were reported by individual patients (Figure 2). In patients who took more than 65% of the drug this inverse relationship between adverse reactions reported and compliance was statistically significant ($r=-0.71$, $p<0.01$; see Figure 3). Compliance was correlated with the duration of infertility ($r=0.44$, $p<0.05$).

Table 3: Adverse reactions reported by 30 patients prescribed 80 μg of ethinyl oestradiol daily.

Symptomatology	No. of individual symptoms	Percentage
Gastrointestinal	37	34.9
Water retention	30	28.3
Gynaecological	26	24.5
Depressed mood	7	6.6
Others:		5.7
Blurred vision	2	
Fatigue	1	
Headache	1	
Vertigo	1	
Breast tension	1	
Total	106	100.0

Table 4: The adverse reactions most frequently reported by 30 patients prescribed 80 μg of oestradiol daily, ranked according to intensity as rated by the patients.

Symptomatology	mild	moderate	severe
Increased vaginal/cervical discharge	10	9	1
Nausea, vomiting	6	7	1
Gastric discomfort, pain	12	2	-
Oedema, gain in weight	9	-	-
Depressed mood	5	1	1
Total	42	19	3

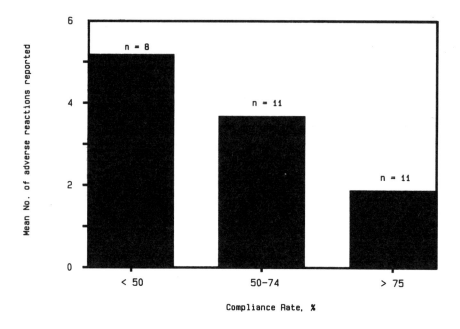

Figure 2: Compliance with 80 µg of ethinyl oestradiol, and adverse reactions reported (SCMPT: sperm-cervical mucus penetration test).

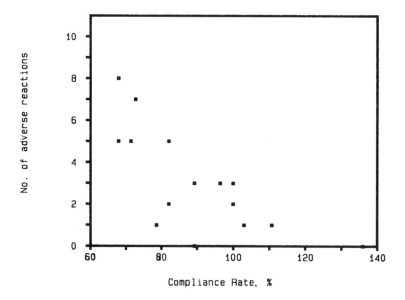

Figure 3: Adverse reactions in 15 compliant patients (compliance >65%).

Comments

Continuous monitoring revealed an average compliance rate of 65% with high-dose ethinyl oestradiol. The patients' adherence to the prescribed QID regimen was poor (<30%). The quality of cervical mucus was high in 29 out of 30 women, regardless of the dose of oestrogens taken. Reports of subjective side effects, mainly of mild intensity, were common (>50%). Compliant patients reported fewer ADRs than less compliant patients.

The question as to the existence of a causal relationship between ADRs and noncompliance with high doses of oestrogens remains unanswered although there was some evidence of an inverse correlation between the compliance rate and the number of ADRs. These findings are far from being generalizable because of the somewhat unusual study setting. However, the setting seemed to be appropriate for the purpose of the study for three reasons. Firstly, the young women of the study population were healthy. Secondly, no patient was on any other pre-scribed drug than ethinyl oestradiol. Therefore, no concomitant medica-tions were likely to interfere with drug compliance or to contribute to adverse reactions. A high compliance rate was assumed as the patients were supposed to be highly motivated. This was confirmed by the association of a higher compliance with longer duration of infertility. The poor adherence to the QID regimen observed is not surprising, how-ever. It compares to results from other studies (Cramer et al., 1989; Brand & Smith, 1974; Gatley, 1968). Finally, adverse effects, if any, were more likely to appear with a high-dose regimen. Actually, in a double blind placebo-controlled study in menopausal women (mean age: 52 years) who were prescribed 75 µg of mestranol daily (Bakke, 1965), the frequency of adverse reactions, as revealed by a questionnaire, was identical (80%) to that found in the present study. Interestingly, the intensity of effects (either desirable or undesirable) did not increase, and no new effects were noted when the dose was doubled.

The following conclusions may carefully be drawn from the present study. The empirically fixed daily dose of 80 µg of ethinyl oestradiol given for 7 days appeared to be too high in regard of the observed dose response, i.e. cervical mucus quality. A dose-finding study, including compliance monitoring, seems to be reasonable. Future studies should also consider employing simpler dosage regimens. The observed association between patients' reports of adverse effects and drug compliance deserves further investigation.

Acknowledgments

We are grateful to Dr. J.-M. Métry and Dr. J. Urquhart (APREX Corp., Fremont, California, U.S.A.) for supplying the compliance monitors and K. Hirschbrunn for excellent help with the manuscript.

References

1. Bakke, J.L. (1965) Pac. Med. Surg. 73, 200-205.

2. Brand, F., Smith, R. (1974) Int. J. Ageing Hum. Dev. 5, 331-346.

3. Cramer, J.A., Mattson, R.H., Prevey, M.L., Scheyer, R.D., and Quellette, B. (1989) J.A.M.A. 261, 3273-3277.

4. Eggert-Kruse, W., Leinhos, G., Gerhard, I., Tilgen, W., and Runnebaum, B. (1989) Fertil. Steril. 51, 317-323.

5. Gatley, M.S. (1968) J. R. Coll. Gen. Pract. 16, 39-44.

6. Haynes, R.B. (1979) In: Compliance in Health Care (R.B. Haynes, D.W. Taylor and D.L. Sackett, Eds). The Johns Hopkins University Press, Baltimore and London, pp. 49-62.

7. Insler, V., Mehmed, H., Eichenbrenner, I., Serr, D.M., and Lunenfeld, B. (1972) Int. J. Gynaecol. Obstet. 10, 223-225.

8. Joyce, C.R.B. (1962) J. Chron. Dis. 15, 1025-1036.

9. Kruse, W. (1988) Abstract, Compliance Monitoring Symposium, sponsored by: Center for the Study of Drug Development, Tufts University, Iselin, New Jersey.

10. Kruse, W., Schierf, G., and Weber, E. (1989) Abstract, Eur. J. Clin. Pharmacol. 36, Suppl. A289.

11. Kruse, W. and Weber, E. (in press) Eur. J. Clin. Pharmacol.

12. Murad, F., and Haynes, Jr. R.C. (1980) In: The Pharmacological Basis of Therapeutics (A. Goodman Gilman, L.S. Goodman, and A. Gilman, Eds), Macmillan Publishing Co., Inc., New York, pp. 1420-1447.

13. Rudd, P., Marshall, G., Taylor, C.B., and Agras, W.S. (1981) Clin. Pharmacol Ther. 29, 278.

14. Spriet, A., and Simon, P. (1985) In: Methodology of clinical drug trials. (A. Spriet and P. Simon, Eds), Karger, Basel-Munich-Paris-London-New York-Dehli-Singapore-Tokyo-Sidney, pp. 138-139.

AAS 29:
Risk Factors for
Adverse Drug Reactions
© 1990 Birkhäuser Verlag Basel

RISK FACTORS AS REFLECTED BY
AN INTENSIVE DRUG MONITORING SYSTEM

T. Jacubeit, D. Drisch and E. Weber

Abstract

Age and gender are often suspected to be risk factors predisposing to ADRs. Therefore the data obtained by the Heidelberg Intensive
Drug Monitoring System were analysed for possible correlations between
these two variables and the incidence of ADRs. Based on the medical
records comprising the time period between 1980 and 1987 information was
available on 70,500 admissions to the Heidelberg University Hospital,
Department of Medicine. Age, gender, number of prescriptions and ADRs
were analysed.

The percentage of patients affected by ADRs rises with advancing age; however the number of prescribed drugs also increases. When the
incidence of ADRs in various age groups was analysed in relation to
prescription data, no effect of age could be found. In contrast there
was a linear correlation between the overall incidence of ADRs (independent of age) and the number of prescriptions per patient (per single admission).

These results clearly document that age does not seem to be
relevant to the incidence of ADRs, but that the risk is related to the
number of drugs prescribed to a particular patient.

Introduction

Several studies have shown the number of adverse drug reactions (ADRs) to increase with age (Hurwitz, 1969a; Klein et al., 1976; Levy et al., 1977; Hoigné et al., 1984). There is no doubt that the increased susceptibility to ADRs observed in elderly patients is due to a number of factors including polymorbidity, alterations in pharmacokinetics and pharmacodynamics and prescription of high-risk medication (Boethius, 1976; Czechanowski et al., 1983; Kruse et al., 1983; Coper & Schulze, 1986; Schwabe & Paffrath, 1988; Jacubeit & Weber, unpublished results). In general, the risk of ADRs clearly increases with the number of medications prescribed (Smith et al., 1966; Kellaway & McCrae, 1973; Steel et al., 1981; Hutchinson et al., 1986). As polypharmacy is extremely common in the elderly, it is still debated whether in these patients age per se or multiple drug prescription is responsible for the high frequency of ADRs observed (Nolan & O'Malley, 1988). Apart from old age, belonging to the female gender has been identified as another important factor which may contribute to ADRs. However, an increased incidence of ADRs in women has not been confirmed unequivocally (Hurwitz, 1969; Klein et al., 1976; Domecq et al., 1980; Williamson & Chopin, 1980; Hoigné et al., 1984; Hutchinson et al., 1986; Jacubeit et al., 1986; Hoigné et al., 1988). Therefore, it seemed worthwhile to evaluate our large ADR data base which was collected by means of an intensive drug monitoring system with particular regard to the impact of age, gender and drug exposure.

Methods

Adverse drug reactions (ADRs) have been assessed in hospitalized patients by means of an intensive drug monitoring system at the department of internal medicine, University of Heidelberg, since 1972. The influence of age, gender and drug exposure on ADRs was studied by evaluating the data collected from 1980 to 1987.

A clinical pharmacologist and a specially trained staff member (from the department of clinical pharmacology) on their twice-weekly ward rounds collected reports on ADRs observed by physicians and/or ward staff. An ADR was defined according to the WHO criteria (World Health Organization, 1969). The procedure used in this drug monitoring system remained unchanged during the entire observation period. Due to the large number of patients surveyed, only severe ADRs were assessed and documented in detail, whereas mild ADRs were recorded "as reported" (Jacubeit et al., 1989). The rate of ADRs that are not detected by the method used appeared to be approximately 50%, irrespective of ADR severity (Fricke et al., 1985).

The present study is based on a total number of 70,407 hospitalizations. In general, more men (57.7%) than women (42.3%) were admitted to this university department of internal medicine. The rate of ADRs, expressed in percent, was calculated according to the number of hospitalizations, patients' age and gender. In addition, ADRs were related to drug exposure (total number of medications prescribed during hospital stay) in a subsample comprising 11,208 hospitalized patients. This sample has been demonstrated to be comparable to the study population as a whole in terms of the distribution of age, gender, drug exposure, length of hospital stay and ADR rate (Käsinger, 1986).

Tables 1a and 1b show the age distribution in the subsample (11,208 patients) and the extent of drug exposure in relation to age, respectively .

Results

In our study population of 70,407 hospitalized patients, a total number of 13,749 ADRs were reported, of which 7,227 occurred in males and 6,522 in females. Admission to hospital was due to an ADR in 1.6% of all hospitalized patients. At least one ADR was reported during hospitalization in 17.9% of all cases, 16.5% in males and 19.9% in females.

The ADR rate increased with age from 8.9% in patients under the age of 19 to more than 20% in patients aged 60 years and over (Figure 1). From the age of 30 upward, the ADR rate consistently remained higher in females than in males. The ADR rate clearly increased with the number of prescribed medications, being 3.2% with 1 to 4 drugs and over 40% with more than 29 prescribed drugs (Figure 2). As can be

T. Jacubeit et al.

Table 1a: Age distribution in the subsample of 11,208 patients.

Patients' age	Number of hospitalizations	Percent
≤49	4,506	40.2
50-59	2,454	21.9
60-69	2,069	18.5
≥70	2,179	19.4
	11,208	100.0

Table 1b: Drug exposure and patients' age.

	Percentage of patients according to age			
Number of medications	≤40	50-59	60-69	≥70
1- 8	51.3	22.6	14.7	11.4
9-16	28.7	22.4	22.8	26.1
17-28	19.2	18.3	24.8	37.7
≥29	15.9	18.0	25.6	40.5

seen from Table 2, this held true irrespective of the patients' age. Patients were divided into three age groups. The increase in the number of prescribed drugs from 1-5 to more than 13 was accompanied by a tenfold increase in the ADR rate. This was found to be the case in young (≤39 yrs), middle-aged (40-59) yrs) and elderly patients (≥60 yrs).

Table 2: Rate of adverse drug reactions (in percent) in relation to age and drug exposure.

	Number of prescribed drugs		
Age (years)	1-5	6-12	13 and more
≤39	2.3	15.1	30.3
40-59	3.9	11.7	30.9
≥60	3.4	11.0	29.8

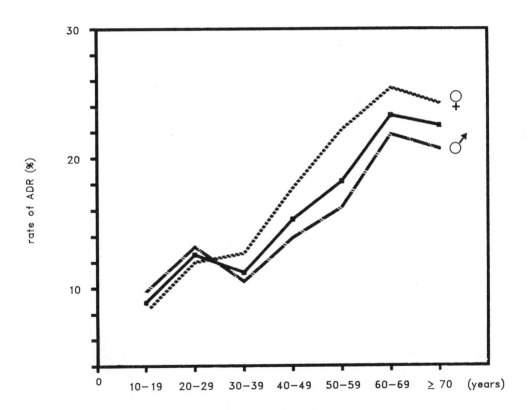

Figure 1: Adverse drug reactions (ADRs) in relation to age and gender.

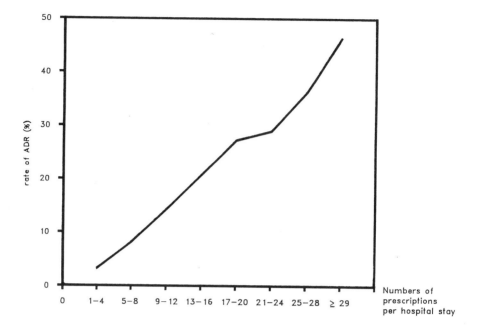

Figure 2:   Adverse drug reactions (ADRs) in relation to   drug exposure.

Discussion

In the present study, the frequency of ADRs was assessed over an eight-year period in 70,407 hospitalized patients by means of an intensive drug monitoring system. Compared with the literature, this patient sample is one of the largest to have been investigated to date (Nolan & O'Malley, 1988). A striking increase in the ADR rate was observed with increasing numbers of prescribed drugs. Reports in the literature and an earlier study, which was conducted in 1975 and employed the same methodology, were confirmed (Smith et al., 1966, Kellaway & McCrae, 1973; Weber et al., 1979; Williamson & Chopin, 1980). In our study population of patients admitted to a university hospital, females appeared to be more susceptible to ADRs than males. This finding represents strong evidence of an increased ADR risk in females (Hurwitz,

1969; Klein et al, 1976; Domecq et al., 1980; Hoigné et al., 1984; Hoigné et al., 1988). In agreement with other investigators' results, we found that the number of ADRs increased with age (Hurwitz 1969a; Klein et al, 1976; Levy et al., 1977; Williamson & Chopin, 1980; Hoigné et al., 1984; Hutchinson et al., 1986). Reports of ADRs were approximately three times as frequent in patients aged 60 years or over than they were in patients under the age of 20. However, relating ADRs to patients' age and drug exposure, there was no substantial difference between the number of ADRs in young and elderly patients. This is in contrast to the findings of Hoigné and co-workers (1984), who reported a significantly higher increase in the ADR rate in patients aged over 60 with prescriptions for more than six medications.

Clearly, the present study has certain limitations, e.g. in that it lacks stratification according to concurrent diseases and their severity. In addition, the symptomatology of drug-induced illness in the elderly may be atypical (Clark & Vestal, 1984). Thus, clear separation of disease-related symptoms from drug-related ones may prove extremely difficult, if not impossible (Nolan & O'Malley, 1988). Furthermore, assessment of the cause-effect relationship between drugs and ADRs is always ambiguous (Karch et al., 1966). Despite the methodology's inherent limitations, the results obtained clearly do not support the assumption that old age per se is a major risk factor for adverse drug reactions. We agree with Vestal and others in our conclusion that polypharmacy has an important impact on unwanted effects; it should definitely be considered more carefully and minimized whenever possible (Royal College of Physicians, 1984; Vestal et al., 1985).

Acknowledgments

We wish to thank all the members of staff at our department of clinical pharmacology who were in various ways involved in this project over the past years. We are particularly indebted to Dr I. Walter-Sack and Dr W. Kruse for their valuable comments on and help with this manuscript. This project received financial support from the Bundesgesundheitsamt and the Bundesverband der pharmazeutischen Industrie e. V.

T. Jacubeit et al.

References

1. Boethius, G. (1976) Acta med. Scand. 202, 241.

2. Clark, B.G., and Vestal, R.E. (1984) Geriatrics 39(2), 53-66.

3. Coper, H., and Schulze, G., (1986) In: Grundlagen der Arzneimittel-
    therapie (W. Dölle, B. Müller-Oehrlinghausen and U. Schwabe, Eds),
    Bibligraphisches Institut, Mannheim, pp. 419-433.

4. Czechanowski, B., Baumann, R., Ding, R., Gundert-Remy, U., Haren-
    berg, J. Hildebrandt, R., von Kaiz-Welle, G., Schaefer, D.O.,
    Spohr, U., Staiger, C., Walter, E., Yakpo-Wempe, C., and Weber, E.
    (1983) Münch. Med. Wschr. 125, 1199-1203.

5. Domecq, C., Naranjo, C.A., Ruiz, I., and Busto, U. (1980) Int. J.
    of Clin. Pharmacol., Ther., and Toxicol. 18, 362-366.

6. Fricke, H., Mayer, I., Meuth, M., Oh, K.-U., Schäfer, D.-O., Ding,
    R., Gemmecke, B., Gundert-Remy, U., Harenberg, J., Kempmann, E.,
    von Kenne, H., Köppenhofer, C., Nador, K., Piper, C., Reindell, K.,
    Schumacher, R., Spohr, U., Staiger, C., and Walter, E. (1985)
    Informationssystem zur Arzneimittelüberwachung - Schwerpunkt uner-
    wünschte Arzneiwirkungen. Bericht über das Forschungsvorhaben DVM
    308, Gesellschaft für Strahlen- und Umweltforschung, München, pp.
    64-84.

7. Hoigné, R., Maurer, P., Maibach, R., Wymann, R., Hess, T., Galeaz-
    zi, R., and Jordi, A. (1988) In: Medical Informatics Europe '88
    (R. Hansen, B.G. Solheim, R.R. O'Moore and F.H. Roger, Eds), Sprin-
    ger, Berlin, Heidelberg, New York, Tokyo, pp. 257-262.

8. Hoigné, R., Sollberger, J., Zoppi, M., Müller, U., Hess, T., Frit-
    schy, D., Stocker, F., and Maibach, R. (1984) Schweiz. med. Wschr.
    114, 1854-1857.

9. Hurwitz, N. (1969) Brit. Med. J. 1, 531-536.

10. Hurwitz, N. (1969a) Br. Med. J. 1, 536.

11. Hutchinson, T.A., Flegel, K.M., Kramer, M.S., Leduc, D.G., and Ho
    Ping Kong, H. (1986) J. Chron. Dis. 39, 533.

12. Jacubeit, T., Auwärter, A., Czechanowski, B., Ding, R., Gutzler,
    F., Henke-Eberhardt, M., Karapanagiotou-Schenkel, I., Kruse, W.,
    Walter-Sack, I., and Weber, E. (1986) Med. Klin. 81, 632-637.

13. Jacubeit, T., Drisch, D., Griffith, D., and Schulte-Bockholt, A.
    (1989) Eur. J. Clin. Pharmacol. 36 (Suppl.), A166.

14. Jacubeit, T., and Weber, E. (unpublished results).

15. Karch, F.E., Smith, C.L., Kerzner, B., Mazzullo, J.M., Weintraub,
    M., and Lasagna, L. (1966) Clin. Pharmacol. Ther. 19, 489-492.

16. Käsinger, W. (1986) Abschätzung des Umfangs von Medikamentenstich-proben und Darstellung an den Daten an der Medizinischen Universi-tätsklinik, doctoral thesis, Heidelberg.

17. Kellaway, G.S.M., and McCrae, E. (1973) N. Z. Med. J. 78, 525.

18. Klein, U., Klein, M., Sturm, H., Rothenbühler, M., Huber, R., Stucki, P., Gikalov, I., Keller, M., and Hoigné, R. (1976) Int. J. Clin. Pharmacol. 13, 187-195.

19. Kruse, W., Mander, T., Merkel, M., Oster, P., and Schlierf, G. (1983) Deutsches Ärzteblatt 80, 27-34.

20. Levy, M., Kletter-Hemo, D., and Nir, I. (1977) Isr. J. Med. Sci. 13, 1065.

21. Nolan, L., and O'Malley, K. (1988) J. Am. Geriatrics Soc. 36, 142-149.

22. Royal College of Physicians (1984) J. R. Coll. Physicians London 18, 7-17.

23. Schwabe, U., and Paffrath, D. (1988) Arzneiverordungsreport '88; Gustav Fischer Verlag, Stuttgart, pp. 377-386.

24. Smith, J.W., Seidl, L.G., and Cluff, L.E. (1966) Ann. Int. Med. 65, 629.

25. Steel, K., Gertman, P.M., and Crescenzi, C. (1981) N. Engl. J. Med. 304, 638.

26. Vestal, R.E., Jue, S.G., and Cusack, B.J. (1985) In: Therapeutics in the elderly (K. O'Malley and J.L. Waddington, Eds), Elsevier Science Publishers B.V., pp. 97-104.

27. Weber, E., Ding, R., Gundert-Remy, U., Harenberg, J., von Kenne, H., Spohr, U., Walter, E., Oh, K.U., Seidel, G., and Fritz, U. (1979) Klinikarzt 8, 851-854.

28. Williamson, J., and Chopin, J.M. (1980) Age and Ageing 9, 73-80.

29. World Health Organization (1969) International drug monitoring, Technical Reports Series, No. 425.

PANEL DISCUSSION

AAS 29:
Risk Factors for
Adverse Drug Reactions
© 1990 Birkhäuser Verlag Basel

PANEL DISCUSSION

Moderator: D. H. Lawson (GB)

Participants: R. Bruppacher (CH), Industry, M. N. G. Dukes (NL),

Academia, and G. R. Venning (GB), Regulatory Authority.

Lawson: Today we have been hearing a lot about risk factors for adverse drug reactions. The objective of our panel discussion is to consider whether we make the correct responses to these risk factors. Given that we have some reasonable information that a drug is associated with an undesirable event, do we have systems in place to ensure that we come to some sort of logical decision on the basis of those risk factors, or do we tend to react in rather illogical ways?

In order to help address this question, I have three very distinguished people on the panel with me. On my right is Dr Rudi Bruppacher, a Swiss citizen, who is head of drug safety with Ciba-Geigy in Bâle and has spent some time in the United States. On my immediate left, there is Graham Dukes, who is head of the regional office for pharmaceuticals with the W.H.O. in Copenhagen and has written several of the "bibles" in this general area. And on his left is Geoffrey Venning, who is a consultant to the pharmaceutical industry, having formerly been a director of research, a medical director with industry, and a senior medical officer in the Department of Health with the regulatory author-ity in the United Kingdom. These people are here wearing their own "personal hats". They are not representing any organization and indeed I have asked them to try and look with a certain bias at the questions that come along. Rudi Bruppacher has been asked to look with a slight bias from the industry point of view, Graham Dukes from the academic point of view, and Geoffrey Venning from the regulatory authority point of view. So, if you feel slightly surprised with some of their responses, that is because I have inserted just a little bias into their responses to ensure an adequate spectrum of comments.

In order to get things going, I would like members of the panel to make a brief statement to start with. Then we have a series of questions that we would like to debate. If anybody has any issues that they would like to bring forward for discussion after the panel have made their preliminary statements would be the time to bring them up. So, perhaps Rudi, could I ask you to start by looking at this whole business of whether we are logical in using our risk factor data?

Bruppacher: O.K., first I think we can fairly state that the pharmaceutical industry has a great interest in identifying risk factors for adverse drug reactions. If we acknowledge the fact that adverse drug reactions do not occur systematically, but occur in certain situations, we have an interest in avoiding these situations in order to avoid unfortunate events and, as for the industry, possible litigation. Our primary aim in industry is to develop safer drugs in the sense of more efficacious drugs or less toxic drugs, possibly even both. This can be achieved through new administration systems, through new chemical substances and so on. More difficult a problem is how we respond to events or to problems that arise when our drugs are then widely used on the market and have left the safe haven of clinical research. How should we deal with the problems then? Many mistakes have been made in the past. It is clear that the industry should respond better in the future. First, it should respond early, it should respond openly but also competently. Now what does "competently" mean? It means that we try to get all the available information and not base our decisions on just one report. Spontaneous reports are often the trigger for such a problem, but we need other sources. We need to go back to old clinical trials; we need to go back to look at the new clinical trials that, most of the time, are going on even with very old drugs; we need to look at intensive monitoring systems such as Professor Hoigné and Ms Jacubeit have shown us, in order to see what those data say; we need to look at postmarketing surveillance systems or prescription-event monitoring systems, usually in a cohort design; we should also look out for the cohort studies that are around, for epidemiological studies and registries. As the two opening papers this morning demonstrated, it has become increasingly important to resort to record-linkage systems in order to see what the problem actually is, how serious it is, how frequently it has occurred and how we have to regard it. And this is where another aspect of the problem comes in. At the time when we need these data, they are available only if we take care that they have been collected in advance. So there is also a need on the part of the industry to ensure that multi-purpose databases are created that can be used to check out difficult situations. I think I will leave it at that for the moment.

Dukes: I will try and make five points very briefly. Firstly, one general point on risk .. It always surprises me that when risk is discussed in relation to a drug, it is often discussed in vacuo without any relationship to all the discussion of efficacy. And yet, some of the drugs which have been in the centre of attention as regards risk are found either to be entirely inefficacious or to be no better than any other drug or to be based on such very poor evidence that one does not know whether they work or not. And if I mention for example the names of dipyrone, and clioquinol, those are drugs where I have found the discussion of risk taking place in vacuo, without looking at the efficacy evidence. Had one looked at it, it might have made the issue much simpler.

Secondly, clearly, when a risk factor appears, one wants to see whether it enables one to limit the risk to a particular group of recipients and then eliminate that group from exposure to the drug. As Dr Bruppacher has said very clearly, right at the start of a drug's career, you often have very poor information; that is true. On the other hand, it is true, also, that drug regulatory authorities - like politicians - often have to take decisions on the basis of incomplete information, because you cannot afford to wait for anything better.

Thirdly, you often can provisionally extrapolate from related drugs, because things are very rarely unique in the drug world. Until you have something better, you may need to extrapolate your warnings, your contraindications, your risk factors from an associated product. What do you actually do with risk data? I just want to mention the fact that it is very easy to say that you introduce a contraindication or

D.H. Lawson et al.

publish a warning. My experience is that people never look at modifications in data sheets or in direction folders. Unless you really hammer
them over the head because the matter is so very important - and it very
rarely is so important that you do that - they will ignore entirely the
fact that a new contraindication or risk factor has appeared. That
applies to doctors and patients alike.

Point four is that once you have a problem with a risk or a
risk factor, go on re-examining the evidence as long as necessary,
because things can change. Look at the oral contraceptives and the way
that some of the warnings developed in the light of risks that apply to
the early high-dose preparations and were automatically adopted into the
directions folders of the later products with much lower oestrogen doses
without even stopping to think whether they still applied or not.

And finally of course, as the Chairman said, do not panic!
There have been some wonderful panics, and to take the case of the oral
contraceptives again, I think Dr Venning and I were both in the industry
making oral contraceptives at the time when the Daily Mirror in London
came out with a headline saying: "Nineteen pills dangerous". At that
particular time, within 48 hours, companies changed their formulations -
mestranol was replaced by oestradiol - and regulatory authorities
accepted the new drugs without any indications as to whether they really
were safer or different from the previous ones. No one really quite knew
what was happening. That was a real old panic.

Venning: It seems to me that risk factors are either identification that
particular patients are more at risk than others - that is to say: age
or sex groups -, that particular indications for a drug carry a greater
risk or that particular dosages and/or durations of the drug are associated with greater risks. So this means that for any drug there are a
number of subgroups of risk category. The evaluation of the risk factors
comes down to detailed evaluation of these different subgroups. Obviously, the response to risk factors must be related to whether the drug has
any benefit in the high-risk group. Many times when drugs have been
taken off the market, it has been because the company did not actually
have good information on the benefit of the drug in different subgroups
of patients. If the company had had accurate and well-documented information, the drug might not have been taken off the market, it might have

132

been restricted to correct indications. Finally, the response of a
company is often inadequate if they do not know how many patients are
using the drug in the different subgroups. Because, at a regulatory
agency, if a drug produces adverse reactions, a common response from the
company is to say: "Oh, but millions of patients have had the drug!".
But, the company is not usually in a position to tell you how many of
those millions had it at such-and-such a dose or for such-and-such a
duration or for such-and-such indications. It would not be difficult for
companies to get this information with a slight modification of their
market research information from organizations like IMS. So, my feeling
is that the best response to the identification of risk factors must be
detailed and accurate collection of data - before the risks emerge - on:
what are the benefits of the drug in the various subgroups which constitute the risk factors?

Lawson: Thank you, gentlemen. Perhaps at this point I should point out
that Geoffrey is acting as an indepentent consultant not to IMS - that
was entirely random that he happened to mention IMS there! I now propose
to consider one or two hypothetical scenarios, but I know that we have
been talking to you, with you and at you all day, so if anyone has a
burning issue that they would like us to be considering this
afternoon? ... Failing that, what I would like to start with is putting
some practical problems to the panel, because I find all those views are
very nice-sounding in theory, but in practice it gets to be a little
more difficult. So, let us pose, for the sake of the argument just now,
that - after a consensus panel had looked at the numbers of case-control
studies and cohort studies on oral contraceptives and breast cancer that
have been conducted in the last little while - we have agreed that there
is a risk ratio of 1.5 for oral contraceptive use amongst subsets of the
population of patients with breast cancer. In particular, it appears
that young women taking long-term oral contraceptives before their
first-term infant are at a higher-than-average risk with a risk ratio of
about 1.5. Given that oral contraceptives seem to protect against
ovarian and endometrial cancer and might also protect against uterine
fibroides, what would the members of the panel think about responding to
this information? Is this a risk ratio that you would like to ignore, or

should we be taking some action, and if so, what action? Who would like to try and tackle that? Rudi ...

Bruppacher: Well, as an epidemiologist I would first say that actions should never be based on risk ratios, but on excess risks. So, what I would recommend is to see what the actual, that is, the added risk with taking oral contraceptives is and to try to estimate what the protective effect is with respect to endometrial cancer, ovarian cancer and other possible effects. I would also include other negative effects that we know of, like thrombo-embolic disease and so on, before then actually trying to formulate a plan of action. So, that is just a methodological remark.

Dukes: Let me take your starting assumption, an increase in the risk of 1.5 in a particular subgroup of the population. That, Chairman, is what you say today. You may say something quite different tomorrow. It is my misfortune to edit the Side Effects of Drug Annual. We have published fourteen of these books so far, and every single volume has said something different about the breast cancer risk, because the evidence has gone up and down and in and out in the period of fifteen years. Now, that is one of the reasons to be extremely cautious about taking decisions on the basis of a figure like that. The other thing, of course, is that you must not look at the figures in isolation. You must look at all the benefits of the pill and all the other types of risk, too, including cardiovascular risks and suchlike and not merely at this particular one.

Lawson: Part of this consensus conference did see data that suggested that there was no overall global increase in the prevalence of breast cancer within the time frame that we were looking at, nor was there evidence of overall increased mortality in the studies that we have been looking at. Does that help us, Geoffrey?

Venning: Well, as far as I know the data indicates that the excess risk for breast cancer in oral contraceptive users is small, the excess reduction in risk for endometrial cancer is small and the excess reduction in risk for ovarian cancer is rather substantial and is many times greater than the risk for breast cancer. Now, how this is dealt with is another matter. One way to answer that question is to give accurate information to patients. The other way to answer it is if in any particular social environment or cultural environment where physicians do not like to give detailed and accurate patient information, they should take their actions based on the good data. But I believe that in the fairly near future there will be a publication doing the arithmetic on these different types of cancer, and the one that sticks out is ovarian cancer.

Lawson: O.K., that gets us a little way down the road. We have got this increased risk ratio that is going to be quoted at us in court when somebody decides to sue the Committee on Safety of Medicines or the B.G.A. for not having taken appropriate action - perhaps the F.D.A. is the one most likely to be sued - but we are proposing to circumvent this by notifying the patients about the risk factor. What are we going to tell them? Because, the data we are basing this information on relates to oral contraceptives that are now not in widespread use, because it takes us so long to get this type of information out, doesn't it, Rudi?

Bruppacher: Well, I think we have a big problem there, not only because of the lack of data but also because of the lack of knowledge about how patients perceive such risk, even if they truly knew it and realized; what does it really matter to them? How do they weigh the benefits against the risks? For instance, a young woman who does not want to get pregnant, how does she weigh that fact against the possibility of having an increased risk of breast cancer in twenty years or so. So, I also think that there is a large field of research that is still open on how patients actually perceive such information. Even if we as physicians believe we are now accurately telling them about the situation and so on, we have only a very slight idea of how patients react to that and what their decisions will be. I think we also need much more of a dialogue with patient groups etc. on these matters. Up to now, such decisions have been made only by experts, and experts, usually, of that specific kind dealing with that risk. They hear oncologists, but I think we should have a much more comprehensive approach which also includes the opinions of those who are possibly involved in the disease.

Lawson: Would you, as a manufacturer of a new low-oestrogen oral contraceptive, like to put a warning on your data sheet about the possibilities of excess risk of breast cancer in previous oral contraceptives with high oestrogen content? What do you think about that?

Bruppacher: I think there is product information and there is general information on treatment. We should not mix them up. I mean, product information has a lot of limitations and requirements placed on it which makes it a special kind of information, but this should not preclude that the general public should be better informed on these risks, not only on a product-specific level, but also in a general way.

Dukes: Does it not depend very much on the type of patient you are dealing with? You have a whole spectrum of patients and the one extreme I can imagine is the patient for whom I would refuse to prescribe an oral contraceptive on the grounds of breast cancer risk. The extreme case would be a woman who herself has had fibroadenosis of the breast, her sister has been operated for breast cancer, her mother died of breast cancer, her own obstetric history is such that it looks as if she might be a high-risk case. Now, that is the one extreme. The other is the woman who has no risk factors at all, where it is hardly even worth talking about the risk of breast cancer. And in between those, there are intermediate situations where you may need to say something, adapt to the individual case. Is that not the way you would react in practice?

Lawson: I think that sounds very reasonable, but the question I was about to ask you as a coauthor of an excellent textbook on medical-legal considerations these days was: what would your coauthor, the one who was the lawyer, think about all of this?

Dukes: Well, there are responsibilities in that particular case at the level of the regulatory authority and the doctor, of course. The regulatory authority has to put information to the doctor and information in a patient package insert which only in the most general terms, I think, would need to talk about this particular type of risk. That would be defensible in the present state of the law in most countries. As far as the doctor is concerned, I think he would be within his rights to behave as I have just described, depending very much on the individual case.

Lawson: Dr Urquhart, can you get yourself to a microphone? You wanted to make a comment.

Urquhart: Well, there are a couple of points which I think are germane to this discussion. One is that the electronic compliance monitoring technique Dr Kruse presented this morning is just now beginning to provide real-time data on patient compliance with oral contraceptives. What that shows is that a substantial minority of women take the oral contraceptives in a way in which they get all the risks but none of the benefits, because they make two-three-day holidays from the regimen, or longer, at critical times in the month when breakthrough ovulation is likely to occur. So, looking ahead, I think that as technology begins to move into the management and reproductive counselling of these patients, that will be a useful method of directing patients towards other methods of contraception if they cannot manage that once-a-day regimen satis-factorily.

The second point is that there is an interesting feature of the American labelling for oral contraceptives which is quite an elaborate risk comparison between the risks of fatality due to various other methods of contraception. It is based on the older data for car-diovascular risk with the oral contraceptives, but it shows in a good context that if a woman decides to give up the use of the oral con-traceptive and switch to another method, she parts with the unique risks of the oral contraceptive, but moves into a new risk spectrum with whatever she does, unless she enters a cloister (and that probably has its unique risks also!). But I think that this question needs to be looked at in a broader context, broader probably than you can encompass within standard labelling, and to say: if you do not use the oral contraceptive then you go to the IUD or you go to a barrier method or something even less effective. Here are the risks that you will encounter because of the relative lack of efficacy of those measures and whatever the pelvic inflammatory disease risks of IUD are etc., etc. So, if you are really going to counsel, if you look at it from a perspective of risk counselling to patients, you have to be prepared to walk through that whole contraceptive choice gauntlet.

Lawson: And first of all we are going to go through that with the doctors, I suspect, the prescribers in the first instance, because not all of them are quite used to handling these sorts of concepts. Geoffrey, before we move on to something else, would you like to wear your regulators hat and say how you reckon you might respond to this problem?

Venning: I think with a regulators hat I would respond by putting out information as accurate as I could and make the company do that. But from the company hat point of view, the company, if it is sensible, will lean over backwards to protect itself against litigation, and it will bend towards disclosing all possible risks.

Lawson: Very good. Well, let us now turn to another topic, because your comments are actually a nice introduction to this. As a clinical pharmacologist, it has always seemed to me that it takes quite a long time to learn how to use drugs properly. There are little subsets of recipients that you have to learn to avoid and so on. One of my great frustrations is that people seem to remove drugs from the market place, either because they are too old (i.e. past patent expiry) before I have learnt how to use them properly or, alternatively, because we now know a little about what adverse effects they produce, so we react in a way that takes them off the market place. Then I have to start learning all over again. For example, I want to quote the nomifensine story here. Here was an antidepressant that was removed from the market place after about eleven years' worth of experience. It was removed on the basis of severe acute haemolytic anaemias occurring after second or subsequent exposure. Now, what I want to ask is: do you, the panel, think that that was a reasonable decision to take, given that the total numbers affected seemed to be very small, or is that a situation where perhaps we should have had warnings rather than removal? And given that we have removal, should we be evaluating the effectiveness of that removal, the cost-benefit, if you like, of removal, which nobody ever seems to do. We talk about cost-benefit in all sorts of other areas, but not in removal of drugs from the market place. What do you think about that? Geoffrey?

Venning: I spoke to Dr Brian Cromey, who happens to be a physician and who was the chairman of Hoechst in the U.K. when this decision was taken. What he tells me is firstly that there was no special benefit that they could advance to justify the use of nomifensine over other similar products. That put them in a difficult position. And the second thing was that - in his judgment - no form of warning was going to protect against the possibility of acute haemolytic anaemia developing and even proving fatal in rather quick time if the warnings were ignored. So, my view, having listened to that side of the story and the fact that it is rather a unique type of adverse reaction occurring only after previous exposure and sensitization, is that here was a me-too drug with no special benefits. It was a correct decision and that nobody has suffered from it because there are other drugs which will act in that way. Now, if in fact there are particular patients who were benefiting from nomifensine more than from other products, Hoechst did not have that information. That was not well documented and was not proven. So, I think if a company wishes to keep products on the market, it should go to considerable lengths to document benefit in different subgroups of patients.

Lawson: So, once you have got your licence, do not go to sleep on your drug! That seems to be the message there. Graham ...

Dukes: Well, I certainly agree with what Geoffrey has been saying about this, but I have a couple of additional things ... Firstly, there is a possibility that, had nomifensine been with us a little longer, it might have turned out to be unique. Its mechanism of action was such that it was hypothesized at that time that it could be a particularly efficient antidepressant in patients with Parkinson's disease. That was never properly examined, because the drug disappeared before the study could be carried out. So we may have lost something useful. The other thing, of course, is that when you talk about the actual number of incidences occurring you have to bear in mind the fact that those reported are only a fraction of those actually taking place. The figures as I recall them were 53 cases of haemolytic anaemia in the U.K. and 400 in the Federal Republic of Germany. Now, Dr Kimble, who runs the adverse reaction monitoring bureau in this country, concludes from his figures that about five percent of adverse reactions get reported. If you look at Professor Stewart Walker's data from Britain, in cases of really serious reactions, about twelve or fifteen percent get reported. So, we may have to increase that number of reports by quite a multiple to find the total number of cases involved. If it were twelve percent, for example, that might mean 3,200 cases in the Federal Republic of Germany. Of those cases, a certain proportion were extremely unpleasant rapid haemolytic anaemias and the patients died. So, there was a certain proportion of cases of rapid death which could not be prevented in the field and, in view of the background which Geoffrey has sketched, I think that the decision was rightly taken.

Lawson: So, we have a nasty problem developing in a drug which seems to be relatively clean over a decade or more. What happens to these people, Rudi? If you are the chap in the firm and you have done the correct thing and you have pulled this drug from the market place, should we be evaluating what happens to these people? Because, if your antidepressants are effective antidepressants, presumably some people might feel pretty depressed after it has been withdrawn and throw themselves into the Neckar or the Rhine or whatever, that is pretty nasty too. Or alternatively, do they go on to the latest antidepressant which your competitor is producing and which of course is pretty clean, because it has only been out for three weeks and we have not had any spontaneous reports of adverse reactions to it at all?

Bruppacher: O.K., let me first comment on one of the remarks Dr Venning made, which is that we should also assemble data on the benefits of our drugs after they have been introduced. The fact is that legal requirements only regard the safety of the drug. The moment the drug is registered it is granted that the drug has at least a potential benefit, so there is little pressure from anybody to go along that way. There are also scientific obstacles to doing it. I mean, the benefit of the drug should be evaluated in the natural environment. That means that it has to be evaluated by means of observational studies. Now, there are many scientists who say that it is impossible to measure intended effects by means of observational studies because of the biases that are inherent in such a design. So, it is very difficult - as regards both the motivation and the scientific possibilities that we have, and in view of the methodological obstacles - to document the benefits of our drugs the same way as we do with the adverse effects. The second thing, of course, is that it is very deplorable that the moment a drug disappears from the market, when there would be a chance of measuring the consequences of such action, there is usually no motivation to do so, either. The manufacturer does not want to throw money after a drug that is lost for him, the regulators can only be proved wrong if it turns out that the effect of the decision was more deleterious than was the drug origi- nally; and of course, the academic people are usually not interested in long-term follow-up studies and have great trouble getting funds for such work. So, to return to your last question, I would say that it is deplorable that the patients who have to be switched to another drug are not followed in a systematic way; there should be a proposal that in such a situation both the regulators and the company should together sponsor a neutral institution to follow up this problem. We have seen some of this in ecological studies, as Feinstein would call them; for instance, recently the declining incidence of Reye's syndrome after the curtailing of the use of aspirin in children was published by the Centers for Disease Control, and so on. But, specificly, I think very little has been done to investigate the effects of regulatory action, and it looks as though in the future, too, very little will be done in that respect.

Lawson: So, maybe we should be setting up multi-purpose databases and anybody who has got any loose money should put it in Gary Friedman's direction, because he is wanting to collect more pharmacy data and presumably therefore would be in a position to answer questions such as the effects of withdrawal, given that the drug was in his market place in the first instance. Perhaps we need more of those types of approach.

Bruppacher: I think there are many others in this room who would also like to help in this respect.

Lawson: Does anybody else want to make a comment about that? A brief comment on that, Dr Urquhart.

Urquhart: Well, following on what Dr Venning said earlier about the need for information on what kind of benefits the drug offers in special groups of patients - Lou Lasagna is not here -, let me make the comment he would make, which is that this is yet another area where we need to give up thinking about herds of patients, group responses, and look at individualized responses and begin to look at the "N-of-one" trial scheme as ways to put on a really objective footing the often-made assertion that there are special groups of patients that got unique benefits from benoxaprofen or this drug or that drug, for which there is never any real hard evidence. But the N-of-one trial formalism, if it had some encouragement from the companies involved, I think, could accumulate data along these lines. And I would like to throw that pot out for critical commentary by others.

Lawson: Brian Strom - do you wish to come in here?

Strom: The N-of-one trial has a major methodological problem in trying to draw out any generalizability. You cannot use the statistics that are used for N-of-one studies, they are in fact invalid. And so, it may be useful to do basically an individual cross-over study to find out if a drug happens to work for an individual patient in a situation when you probably can tell any way, without the formality of the N-of-one trial. But to try to use one patient or a few isolated patients to decide whether or not a drug works on a general scale is really inappropriate. What I would propose is another alternative, in answer again to Rudi's suggestion about studying efficacy after marketing with the limitations of nonexperimental techniques. There are ways of doing postmarketing randomized clinical trials which can be done with the cost of a post-marketing study but yet use randomization, take advantage of the fact that the drugs are already marketed and have, for example, people pre-scribe study drug and then follow the patient in the usual way. You would be blinded; you are not asking the physician to do do anything more than you normally would do. It is a natural setting; you take advantage of the medical records as they exist. You do not have to pay the physician 3,000 dollars per patient, because you are not asking him to do anything more than he otherwise would do. And yet you have the elegance of the randomized trial, without the cost and artificiality.

So, there are other approaches, but yet people are very reluctant to try to test them or use them.

Lawson: It seems to me that one of the problems we have is that the effective patent life of drugs is now getting so short that people do not want to indulge in that sort of study just now. But I will leave that one to hang in the air and see if anybody plucks it out later. Let us go on now and think about Brian Strom's presentation this morning, because he was covering a big area that has caused quite a lot of concern over the years, namely concern about serious GI bleeding and about death in the elderly taking non-steroidal anti-inflammatory drugs. What I want to question the panel about is: do we pay enough attention to the benefits of non-steroidals in the elderly and maybe quality of life? Is death the right end point to look at, therefore, or should we be looking at "quality of life" and are we, in fact, paying a fair price for the rather indiscriminate use patterns that have developed in non-steroidals over the years? Who would like to rise to that one?

Bruppacher: Well, firstly we have to say that here we are in the dilemma that the major risk factor age is also the major determinant for the need of the drug. So you get much higher usage in these age groups, because they also need it more and it is even more important for them to stay mobile at an older age. So, this is a problem that is very hard to solve, and judgment has to be made on the value of symptomatic relief of diseased states and the possible reduction in length of life. I do not think we can avoid setting up such studies.

Lawson: In industry, or in general?

Bruppacher: No, I would say this is in general. Also, I should not like to forget to say that, of course, precautions could be taken that would probably reduce the risk in elderly people by avoiding use of non-steroidal anti-inflammatory drugs in patients with known active ulcers etc.

Lawson: We have already heard that one of the ways to reduce the risk in elderly people is not to give them the drugs. That is the general message of clinical pharmacology. Lie down and let the feeling wear off rather than prescribe for certain populations. Often the patient benefits from that approach Perhaps some of the elderly who die are people who do not actually need to take the non-steroidals, maybe the total numbers who are having GI bleeds could be reduced by more rational prescribing?

Bruppacher: Well, may I again come back to the fact that we must mention other factors, such as alcohol; I agree that of course only a drug with a good indication is a useful drug, and as we have also seen from the paper by, I think, Dr Kruse, it is very often that we have the suspicion that the adverse drug reactions are even more frequent when the drug is not used properly or it is not indicated. This is certainly the first point that should be respected, that is only to give the drug to those who actually can profit from it. But again, perhaps by cutting down on other risk factors, the overall risk of bleeding and perforated peptic ulcer could also be reduced in this population, even though some of the studies show that in the very old age group the two lines come together again. So it does not really matter; there is a very high risk for everybody of that age.

Lawson: If you live that long, the physicians will not kill you, yes. Graham?

Dukes: Well, Chairman, I would have thought that society had accomodated this particular problem pretty well, realizing that these drugs are necessary and going on using them in spite of the problems. People know that there is a low level of constant bleeding in many users of these drugs and they check on the possibility of anaemia now and again in elderly patients, quite apart from being prepared for a severe bleed if it occurs. But I do not think any of these drugs have been taken off the market because of gastrointestinal problems. Those that have disappeared have done so for quite different reasons; benoxaprofen, for example, because of problems with the liver and the skin, and one or two other drugs for anaphylactic reactions and suchlike, but not because of gastrointestinal problems.

Lawson: Geoffrey?

Venning: I think, with the wisdom of hindsight, regulatory agencies, particularly the C.S.M. in my country, licensed too many non-steroidal anti-inflammatories, and with a harder look at the data on benefit and on getting the dose right, some of these problems would have been avoided. I would have thought that a harder line from the regulatory agencies would probably have saved a lot of elderly people's lives.

Lawson: Certainly regulatory agencies seem to be taking a slightly harder line these days. Most people who are employed by drug firms that are looking to get a new non-steroidal anti-inflammatory agent registered are tending also to look at the situation's vacant column in the papers on the ground that their pension might not be greatly enhanced by the enthusiasm of the C.S.M. or F.D.A. for their new drug. Brian, do you want to come in here?

Strom: My sense is: what generally causes the loss of a drug, as Dr Dukes said, usually is not something like GI bleeding, though osmosin was an exception, but is generally a much less common but serious idiosyncratic reaction, particularly in a setting where there are lots of other alternatives, so that, unless a drug has a unique benefit, a unique problem is a reason for removal. One not only has to take into account risk versus benefit for that drug, but risk versus other alternative treatments.

Dukes: Yes, osmosin was an exception. But, osmosin was almost custom-built to provide a borehole in the intestine. It was not a typical case, I think.

Lawson: Professor Velo.

Velo: I should like to go back to the point Dr Venning made, which was: do you really need such numbers of non-steroidal anti-inflammatory drugs? My point is now that it would be much better in my opinion to undertake good studies of the efficacy and the toxicity of a few non-steroidal anti-inflammatory drugs and to avoid the big confusion with such large numbers of NSAIDs. I should like to ask the panel what they think about this.

Lawson: Non-steroidals, too many me-too drugs? Rudi!

Bruppacher: O.K., it is not only because I am supposed to speak for the industry here that I strongly believe that it is good to have so many of them around, especially because none of them is perfect. If you have ever seen arthritic patients going on for a long time with these drugs, you often see them start with a drug. At first and they are quite satisfied with the drug, then after a while they get dissatisfied. You can switch them to another drug and they improve again. Actually the patient seems to be benefited by the change, especially if there are different types of chemical substances which you can assume to have a different metabolism and slightly different treatment properties which you can utilize. Individual patients sometimes react very differently even to slight modification of drugs, so I am in favour of diversity here.

Lawson: Let me ask you then, Geoffrey. In the new, magnificent one-state drug regulatory authority that is going to take over when the E.E.C. really gets into swing, would they like a "need" clause in as well as a "safety, quality and efficacy" clause with regard to new drug applications? Geoffrey ...

Venning: Well, the only country that has a need clause is Norway, and I think before getting a need clause, the E.E.C. wants to catch up with the F.D.A. and get the dose right for new drugs. The F.D.A. requires that the dose proposed should be needed, and that, I would say, is absolutely essential. I think to move on to a need clause in the other sense is a political issue, rather than a pharmacological one.

Lawson: Indeed, highly political. Graham ...

Dukes: When the W.H.O. looked at this specific issue a few years ago - the figures are a little out of date - there were, in Britain and Holland, twenty-five drugs of this type on the market. There were sixty in Italy and there were seven in Norway. - Norway had the need clause. - Now, when we looked at the drugs that you actually needed to cover the market, the Norwegians did not have enough drugs on the market. To cover the spectrum of effect you probably require ten or twelve or something like that. So, the twenty-five is not excessive; the sixty is surely rather confusing.

Lawson: Now, of course, the other thing to keep in mind is that the Norwegians do not have an indigenous pharmaceutical industry, whereas the new Common Market is certainly going to have a big pharmaceutical industry. O.K, Dr Urquhart, one brief comment. I want to touch one other topic before it is time for the boat to go.

Urquhart: G.D. Searle have just introduced, in the United States, a product that is designed to be the antidote for the problems of NSAID-induced bleeding we have been discussing. However, they seem to have had some problems in gaining physician acceptance of it. I wonder, does the panel have any words of wisdom as to how that antidote should be directed in terms of which patients receiving NSAIDs should receive misoprostil?

Lawson: O.K., Graham, do you think we should routinely be prescribing for everybody a drug which might be beneficial in preventing an adverse reaction that may occur in an unpredictable member of the community that is receiving another drug?

Dukes: No. Quite simply, you end up with polypharmacy.

Bruppacher: I would also say no.

Venning: I would say no, too.

Lawson: Nobody is keen on that approach. O.K. Let me just perhaps finish by saying that earlier on today I had to wear my Malcolm-Lader hat, for which I apologize, but Malcolm was going to speak about "addictive risks" with benzodiazepines, which of course is causing a big anxiety just now. I wonder whether the members of the panel with their years of experience behind them regard this as a major problem. Do you think it is a major benzodiazepine problem, or is it a problem that people who are desperate to be addicted to something or other happen to get hooked on benzodiazepines? Who is going to tackle that one?

147

Dukes: Any useful tool that you create in society, whether it be a motorcycle or electricity supply, will be misused by someone. Any drug that will protect from anxiety will be so attractive by protecting from anxiety that it will be overused. It will give people that comforting cocoon of being shielded away from society's problems. So, even if there was no real risk of dependence with the benzodiazepines, they would be overused. The solution here lies not with controls on the drugs. We are not concerned with the drugs; we are concerned with the way that they are used and misused, with the whole question of the doctor's and the patient's attitude to these things.

Bruppacher: May I add to that? It is a tragedy that - you mentioned barbiturates, thalidomide and benzodiazepines this morning - the safer a drug becomes, the more likely it is to be abused, because people are not so afraid of it any more. Not only the patients, but of course also the physicians. And some of the progress that one makes in producing a safer drug is, so to speak, eaten away by the subsequent reaction of the public who say: "Now we have something safe, so we can also use it in this situation, we do not have to be so careful." So, this reinforces what Professor Dukes said.

Lawson: Geoffrey ...

Venning: Well, I just do not have the data. I do not know whether the people on benzodiazepines take more or less alcohol and whether they take more or less alcohol when they stop. So, I do not think I can answer this question; I would like to see the data.

Lawson: O.K., Ladies and Gentlemen, does anybody want to make any comments about addiction and benzodiazepines? ... No. Well, we will keep a very closeful eye on your habits this evening on the boat and make sure that none of you become unduly addicted to eating and drinking during the boat trip. In the meantime I should like now to bring this panel discussion to a close. I do not think we have solved problems, but we have certainly aired quite a few this afternoon. I would like to thank the members for their participation.

Also, I am told I have to draw this symposium to a close. In doing so I would like to thank the people who have been doing all the organizing. The symposium has gone superbly well thanks to their efforts. Secondly, on behalf of Professor Hoigné and myself, and I am sure on behalf of the audience, too, I would like to thank Dr Walter-Sack and Professor Weber for doing most of the work here. Because, it is somewhat ironic that Professor Hoigné's name and mine are on the front of the programme here when in fact, we came along here briefly to draw up the basic framework, and then the next thing that happened was that we came here to this excellent symposium. Really, Professor Weber and Dr Walter-Sack are the two people who have put in an enormous amount of effort to get the meeting off the ground, and I would like to thank them publicly and I hope you will all join with me in thanking them for their efforts on your behalf.

AGENTS AND ACTIONS SUPPLEMENTS

Edited by K. Brune

AAS 1
Proceedings of the Symposium
on Aspirin and Related Drugs:
Their Actions und Uses
Edited by K.D. Rainsford,
K. Brune, M.W. Whitehouse.
ISBN 3-7643-0902-4

AAS 2
Recent Developments in the
Pharmacology of Inflammatory
Mediators
Proceedings of an International
Symposium held in Rotterdam,
under auspices of the Dutch
Society for Physiology and
Pharmacology, in November 1976
Edited by I.L. Bonta.
ISBN 3-7643-0914-8

AAS 3
Inflammation: Mechanisms and
their Impact on Therapy
Proceedings of an Advanced
Teaching Course held in
Rotterdam, November 1976
Edited by I.L. Bonta,
J. Thompson, K. Brune.
ISBN 3-7643-0913-X

AAS 5
Connective Tissue Changes in
Rheumatoid Arthritis and the
Use of Penicillamine
Proceedings of a Review
Symposium held in Rotterdam,
9-10 March 1979, under the
auspices of the ¨Gerrit Jan
Mulder Foundation¨
Edited by I.L. Bonta, A. Cats.
ISBN 3-7643-1127-4

AAS 6
Prostaglandins and Inflammation
Proceedings of an International
Conference, Kings College,
Hospital Medical School, London
August 1979.
Edited by K. Rainsford,
A.W. Ford-Hutchinson.
ISBN 3-7643-1132-0

AAS 7
Trends in Inflammation
Research 1
Proceedings of the International
Meeting on Inflammation at
Verona, September 24-27, 1979.
Edited by G.P. Velo.
ISBN 3-7643-1177-0

AAS 8
Trace Elements in the
Pathogenesis and Treatment of
Inflammation
Edited by K.D. Rainsford,
K. Brune, M.W. Whitehouse.
ISBN 3-7643-1201-7

AAS 9
Recent Progress on Kinins
Proceedings of the International
Conference ¨Kinin 81-Munich¨,
Munich, Nov. 2-5, 1981.
Edited by H. Fritz, G. Dietze,
F. Fiedler, G.L. Haberland.
ISBN 3-7643-1324-2

AAS 10
Trends in Inflammation
Research 2
Pharmacology, Biochemistry
and Immunology 4th Summer
Colloquium on Pharmacology,
Biochemistry and Immunology
of Inflammation,
Martin-Luther-University,
Halle-Wittenberg, July 1, 1981.
Edited by H. Bekemeier,
R. Hirschelmann.
ISBN 3-7643-1344-7

AAS 11
Cologne Atherosclerosis
Conference
Proceedings of the Cologne
Atherosclerosis Conference,
May 1982.
Edited by M.J. Parnham,
J. Winkelmann.
ISBN 3-7643-1325-0

AAS 12
Leukocyte Locomotion and
Chemotaxis
Proceedings of the 1st
International Conference on
Leukocyte Locomotion and
Chemotaxis, Gersau,
May 16-21, 1982.
Edited by H.U. Keller,
G.O. Till.
ISBN 3-7643-1489-3

AAS 13
Pharmacology of Asthma
Proceedings of a Workshop
at the Cardiothoracic
Institute,
London, March 16-17, 1982.
Edited by K.D. Rainsford,
J. Morley.
ISBN 3-7643-1503-2

AAS 14
Pathophysiology and Treatment of
Asthma and Arthritis
Symposium held at the Erasmus
University,
Rotterdam, October 14-15, 1982,
to celebrate the 60th birthday
of Prof. Dr. I.L. Bonta.
Edited by P.R. Saxena,
G.R. Elliott.
ISBN 3-7643-1628-4

AAS 15
Ticlopidine: Quo Vadis?
Edited by J.L. Gordon.
ISBN 3-7643-1632-2

AAS 16
Cologne Atherosclerosis
Conference No. 2: Lipids
2nd Cologne Atherosclerosis
Conference, Cologne,
May 2-4, 1984.
Edited by M.J. Parnham.
ISBN 3-7643-1645-4

AAS 17
Non-Steroidal
Anti-Inflammatory Drugs
Proceedings of a Symposium at
Leura, New South Wales,
Australia, May 16-18, 1985.
Edited by Peter Brooks,
Richard Day.
ISBN 3-7642-1750-7

AAS 18
Recent Advances in Connective
Tissue Research
Selected Papers of a
Symposium held at Salamander
Bay, Port Stephens, N.S.W.,
Australia, May 26-29, 1985.
Edited by Peter Gosh.
ISBN 3-7643-1775-2

AAS 19
100 Years of Pyrazolone Drugs
An Update
Edited by Kay Brune.
ISBN 3-7643-1814-7

AAS 20
Cologne Atherosclerosis
Conference No. 3: Platelets
3rd Cologne
Atherosclerosis Conference,
Cologne, April 23-25, 1986.
Edited by M.J. Parnham.
ISBN 3-7643-1805-8

AAS 21
PAF, Platelets, and Asthma
Edited by
M. Schmitz-Schumann,
G. Menz, C.P. Page.
1987, 264 pages, Hardcover
ISBN 3-7643-1806-6

AAS 22
Vasodepressor Hormones in
Hypertension Prostaglandins and
Kallikrein-Kinins
Edited by G. Bönner,
O.A. Carretero, H. Küppers,
J.C. McGiff.
1987. 370 pages, Hardcover
ISBN 3-7643-1922-4

AAS 23
Directions for New Anti-Asthma
Drugs
Proceedings of a Satellite
Meeting of the Xth International
Congress of Pharmacology
Edited by S. O'Donnell,
C.G.A. Persson.
ISBN 3-7643-1957-7

AAS 24
Basis for Variability of
Response to Anti-Rheumatic Drugs
Proceedings of a Satellite
Meeting of the Xth International
Congress of Pharmacology
Edited by P.M. Brooks, R.O. Day,
K. Williams, G. Graham.
ISBN 3-7643-1959-3

AAS 25
Non-Opioid (OTC)
Analgesics - Risks/Benefits in
Perspective
Edited by K. Brune.
ISBN 3-7643-2251-9

AAS 26
Cologne Atherosclerosis Conference
No. 4: Cholesterol-Homeostasis
Edited by M.J. Parnham, R. Niemann.
ISBN 3-7643-2247-0

AAS 27
Anti-Inflammatory Drugs from Plant
and Marine Sources
Edited by D.A. Lewis.
ISBN 3-7643-2265-9

AAS 28
Intrinsic Asthma
Edited by M. Schmitz-Schumann,
G. Menz, U. Costabel, C.P. Page.
ISBN 3-7643-2289-6

Birkhäuser
Verlag
Basel·Boston·Berlin